MARKETING

MATTERS

A Guide for Healthcare Executives

MARKETING

MATTERS

A Guide for Healthcare Executives

Richard K. Thomas

Michael Calhoun

ACHE Management Series

Health Administration Press

Your board, staff, or clients may also benefit from this book's insight. For more information on quantity discounts, contact the Health Administration Press Marketing Manager at (312) 424-9470.

This publication is intended to provide accurate and authoritative information in regard to the subject matter covered. It is sold, or otherwise provided, with the understanding that the publisher is not engaged in rendering professional services. If professional advice or other expert assistance is required, the services of a competent professional should be sought.

The statements and opinions contained in this book are strictly those of the author and do not represent the official positions of the American College of Healthcare Executives or of the Foundation of the American College of Healthcare Executives.

11 10 09 08 07   5 4 3 2 1

Library of Congress Cataloging-in-Publication Data

Thomas, Richard K., 1944-
   Marketing matters : a guide for healthcare executives / Richard K. Thomas, Michael Calhoun.
      p. cm.
   Includes bibliographical references.
   ISBN-13: 978-1-56793-276-8
   ISBN-10: 1-56793-276-2 (alk. paper)
   1. Medical care—Marketing. 2. Hospital care—Marketing. I. Calhoun, Michael, 1949-
II. Title

RA410.56 .T49 2007
362.1068'8—dc22   2007060370

The paper used in this publication meets the minimum requirements of American National Standard for Information Sciences—Permanence of Paper for Printed Library Materials, ANSI Z39.48-1984. ∞ ™

Acquisitions editor: Audrey Kaufman; Project manager: Gregory Sebben;
Layout editor and cover designer: Chris Underdown

Health Administration Press
A division of the Foundation of the
   American College of Healthcare Executives
1 North Franklin Street, Suite 1700
Chicago, IL 60606-3529
(312) 424-2800

Contents

Foreword

As a hospital administrator beginning my career in the early 1960s, I have witnessed the emergence and subsequent maturation of healthcare marketing. When I began my career there were few for-profit hospitals and most major hospitals were church sponsored. There were few constraints on the utilization of health services and few hospitals thought in terms of competing for patients. Healthcare administrators were not exposed to marketing on the job or in their educational curricula.

As a young administrator for a major health system I became (mostly by default) the person in my organization that interacted with members of the news media. The task of publishing a monthly employee newsletter was added to this responsibility. By performing these roles I was able to develop an appreciation for the marketing function early in my career. I even found myself in the unique position of announcing the death of Elvis Presley to the public and managing the understandable attention the hospital received from the international media.

With the enactment of Medicare legislation in 1965, the new reimbursement formula provided for-profit hospitals with a predictable return on investment. This created an incentive for growth and consolidation in the for-profit sector. Not-for-profit hospitals—many of which had longstanding monopolies within their service areas—saw this development as a real threat.

At the same time, the unrestrained increase in hospital costs encouraged the emergence of managed care. This, in turn, resulted in a dramatic shift from inpatient care to outpatient care. All of a sudden, hospitals had to openly compete for patients. This new competitive environment in healthcare demanded the adoption of marketing on the part of healthcare organizations in order to survive.

Initially, hospitals put up considerable resistance to formal marketing programs. Most hospital administrators felt they were on a mission—reflecting their religious affiliation. Physicians were particularly opposed to the use of marketing, believing self-promotion to be unprofessional and unethical. This negative attitude toward marketing gradually changed as competition intensified and marketing came to be accepted as an integral function of hospitals.

Hospital executives eventually came to appreciate the ability of marketing to profile their customers, identify their organization's strengths and weaknesses, strengthen their organization's strategic plan, and more effectively communicate with the communities they serve as well as their employees and their medical staffs.

Richard K. Thomas and Michael Calhoun have collaborated in the presentation of an in-depth depiction of marketing for today's healthcare administrator. I worked with both Rick and Mike for several years in a not-for-profit, multi-hospital system. Rick was an experienced market research professional and Mike brought marketing experience to bear from other industries to healthcare, resulting in the organization's first formal marketing program.

This book, *Marketing Matters: A Guide for Healthcare Executives*, does an outstanding job of explaining all aspects of an effective marketing program. They clearly review the value of marketing, explain how that value can be measured, and demonstrate how marketing can be used to enhance the performance of a healthcare organization.

Without a doubt, this book will provide any health professional with a better understanding of the marketing function in healthcare and a greater appreciation of the contribution that marketing can make to any healthcare organization.

—Maurice Elliott, CEO Emeritus
Methodist Healthcare
Memphis, Tennessee

Preface

Most observers of the marketing phenomenon in healthcare pinpoint the mid-1970s for the emergence of healthcare marketing as a separate discipline. While formal marketing activities among retail-oriented healthcare organizations (i.e., health insurance, pharmaceuticals, medical supplies) became common early on, health services providers had long resisted incorporating formal marketing activities into their operations. Of course, hospitals and other healthcare organizations were "marketing" under the guise of public relations, physician relationship development, community services, and other activities, but few health professionals equated these efforts with true marketing.

In the 1980s, the formal recognition of marketing as an appropriate activity for health services providers represented an important milestone. It led to the establishment of marketing budgets and the creation of numerous new positions within healthcare organizations, culminating with the establishment of the position of vice president for marketing in many organizations. This development opened healthcare up to an influx of concepts and methods from other industries and helped foster the introduction of modern business practices into the healthcare arena.

Most would agree that, after years of grudging acceptance, marketing has become reasonably well established as a legitimate function in healthcare. The industry has demonstrated surges of interest in marketing, followed by periods of retrenchment when marketing—and marketers—were considered unnecessary and/or inappropriate. Periods of prosperity for marketing have alternated with periods of neglect over the past 25 years. There have been periods of almost reckless marketing frenzy, periods of hasty retreat, and an ongoing tension between those who eagerly accepted marketing as a function of the healthcare organization and those who doggedly resisted its intrusion into their realm.

By the early 1990s, healthcare executives recognized that marketing did not consist of spending large amounts of money on mass media advertising. Progressive organizations began to assess their marketing objectives in a more reasonable light. They tried to understand the market, their customers, and their customers' motivations. Marketers, too, had learned some important lessons. Few marketing techniques could be transferred unmodified from other industries. The messages and the methods had to be tailored to healthcare. Sensitive issues that are not factors in other industries had to be addressed in a healthcare context. Further, marketers realized they were faced with unique situations in healthcare that existed in no other industry.

Today, healthcare is still struggling to find the appropriate role for marketing, and marketers continue to search for their niche within healthcare. As the future dawns, however, marketing appears poised to play a greater role in the new healthcare environment. A core of professional healthcare marketers has emerged with a much better understanding of the market and their customers. They are applying increasingly sophisticated market research techniques. They have developed an appreciation for what works and does not work in terms of marketing initiatives and have crafted new techniques specifically for the healthcare market. These are encouraging developments given the fact that virtually every trend in healthcare points to the need for effective marketing capabilities.

The objective of this book is to allow you—the healthcare executive—to benefit from a quarter century of fits and starts in healthcare marketing. We hope to distill those kernels of marketing wisdom and lore as well as the developments appearing on the horizon that will prepare you for the exigencies of today's—and tomorrow's—healthcare environment.

Acknowledgments

The authors would like to acknowledge the numerous colleagues who served as mentors and provided inspiration. Richard Thomas would particularly like to thank the staff of the American Marketing Association for the opportunities provided him through the editorship of Marketing Health Services. Michael Calhoun would like to express his heartfelt thanks to Merrie Spaeth of Spaeth Communications. Her devotion to the nuances of business communication and her groundbreaking and backbreaking work on what people hear, what they believe, and what they remember are reflected throughout the material presented here.

CHAPTER 1

An Introduction to Healthcare Marketing

WHAT IS HEALTHCARE MARKETING AND WHY IS IT IMPORTANT TODAY?

Why should a healthcare executive be concerned with marketing? Aside from making sure that the organization is running smoothly, perhaps nothing is as important to the organization in today's healthcare environment as marketing. Virtually all of the trends affecting healthcare today—as well as those predicted for the future—underscore the importance of marketing. With the rise of consumerism, increasing competition, thinner margins, and changing payer mix, the implications for marketing are clear: the successful healthcare organization will be a "marketing organization."

What do we really mean by "marketing"? Marketing in its simplest form is nothing more than reputation management. However, we will see that "nothing more" covers a lot of territory. The biggest single hurdle yet to be overcome in the marketing profession is the gap between what many healthcare executives think marketing is, what it really is, and how they can best take advantage of the marketing process. To successfully market any healthcare organization, you must believe two things: *A carefully managed reputation is better than an unmanaged one,* and *disciplined consistency is better than inconsistency.* Much of what follows in this book underscores these two points.

More than most other aspects of healthcare administration, "context" is especially important for marketing. Much of this context has to do with the market itself. Geography, population, competition, stakeholders, and budgets are all factors that make up about half of the marketing context. The other half of the context exists within the minds of consumers. What they think we are, what they believe, and what they remember about us *is* the marketing reality. Things are happening in the mind of the consumer whether you participate in the process or not.

WHY SHOULD YOU MARKET?

The healthcare executive needs to consider why she is marketing, and this "why" should be quantifiable. The reflex answer might be that the organization needs to sell something. The need to sell something is seldom actually (or at least solely) the reason for marketing in healthcare, and a number of factors—some positive, some negative—might serve to initiate a marketing campaign. You might initiate marketing activities

- to reach a specific goal;
- to support a broad organizational strategy; or
- to respond to identified needs, deficiencies, or changing market conditions, possibly as a result of research.

Often, however, the factors that drive a marketing initiative are less positive. Sometimes a healthcare executive may believe a marketing campaign is the only way to address a problem, or he may simply be following someone else's advice when someone tells him marketing is important. All too often, healthcare organizations undertake marketing campaigns because the competition is doing it, or in an attempt to raise the prestige of the organization. Sometimes marketing represents an attempt to create a positive (and perhaps misleading) image to offset a deficiency or an adverse event. When marketing goes wrong in healthcare, it is usually because the initiative was launched for the wrong reason.

What, then, are the "right" reasons for marketing in healthcare?

Building Awareness

With the introduction of new products and the emergence of an informed consumer, healthcare organizations must build awareness of their services and expose target audiences to their capabilities. The attention span of the healthcare consumer is short, and the public must be continuously reminded of the organization's availability.

Enhancing Visibility or Image

With the increasing standardization of healthcare services and a growing appreciation of "reputation," healthcare organizations find it necessary to initiate marketing campaigns that improve top-of-mind awareness and distinguish them from their competitors. Consumers need to know how your organization is different and why they should care.

Improving Market Penetration

Healthcare organizations faced with growing competition can use marketing as a means of increasing patient volumes, improving revenues, and gaining market share. With few new patients in many markets, marketing becomes critical for retaining existing customers and attracting competitors' customers. You don't want consumers choosing just any health service, you want them to choose *your* health service.

Serving as an Information Resource

Healthcare organizations are considered an important resource for the community. Marketing serves not only the need to make consumers aware of *your* services, but it also fulfills your responsibility to educate the community with regard to positive health behavior. In community after community, the most trusted healthcare organizations are those that are perceived as reliable sources of health information.

Influencing Consumer Decision Making

Once marketers realized that the consumer plays a part in healthcare decision making, they recognized the role of marketing in influencing that decision making. By convincing consumers to decide on a particular organization's services and to more effectively use the healthcare system, marketing should be a force for the creation of consumer demand and the subsequent channeling of that demand.

Offsetting Competitive Marketing

Once healthcare organizations realized that their competitors were adopting aggressive marketing approaches, they began to adopt a stance of defensive marketing. While getting involved in "marketing wars" is not recommended, taking an aggressive approach to establishing a position in the market is both reasonable and desirable.

Creating an Internal "Sales Force"

The forgotten audience for an organization's marketing efforts is often its own employees. Healthcare organizations can establish a marketing mindset among their employees via internal marketing, thereby turning every associate into a "salesperson" and creating a "marketing organization."

Attracting Medical Staff and Employees

As the healthcare industry has expanded, competition for skilled workers has increased. Hospitals and other healthcare providers find it necessary to promote themselves to potential employees by marketing the superior benefits that they offer to recruits.

WHAT HAVE WE LEARNED ABOUT MARKETING?

Until recently, healthcare administration education programs did not actively teach healthcare marketing to their students, and the expertise needed to expand the profession and add value to the organization was best provided by those with experience in the field—those who learned firsthand how to apply the tools of the marketing trade to the healthcare arena. Here are some conclusions based on the experiences of those who pioneered the field.

Every Organization Has a Reputation, Whether They Want One or Not

There are no empty spaces in people's consciousness; if they are aware of you, you have been assigned a reputation, even if by default.

While your organization may occupy a position in the market based on statistics, you also have a position in the market in the mind of the consumer. The more control you exercise over this reputation, the more favorably your organization will be perceived.

Default Reputations Are Almost Always Negative

For some reason, negative news seems easier to remember. In an environment that has become increasingly distrustful of physicians and hospitals and rife with recurring news stories on medical errors and the perpetration of fraud by healthcare organizations, not being counted as one of "them" is most preferable. By proactively controlling your perception in the community, you can reinforce a positive reputation.

If You Create, Nourish, Grow, and Protect Your Reputation, You Can Implant It in the Mind of the Marketplace

Three factors are at work: What people hear, what they believe, and what they remember. A reputation must be positive and appropriate for the institution and the specific marketplace in which it operates. It must also be believable and credible, and it absolutely must be repeated at every opportunity.

Having a Good Reputation Will Increase Income and Retain Business, Especially if You Can Internalize It

When every employee of the organization knows what their marketing reputation is, and that they must personally deliver on that reputation every single day, it's amazing how well people respond and how the business prospers. Obviously, a bad reputation will have the opposite effect.

It's Easier (and Cheaper) to Stay Out of Trouble Than to Get Out of Trouble

Because of the way in which healthcare is perceived, a few adverse events can easily color everyone's perception of the organization. There are numerous stories of how prestigious institutions suffered a serious public relations (PR) blow as the result of a clinical error. Although adverse events cannot always be avoided, we would argue that marketing organizations are more diligent in this regard. A proactive marketing approach that is sensitive to the community being served can go a long way toward defusing any negative fallout.

WHEN SHOULD YOU MARKET?

In healthcare, marketing activity is often associated with the introduction of a new service or the sponsorship of some "event." But true marketing is not something that starts and stops in response to short-term developments. Rather, it is an ongoing process that reflects the strategic direction of the organization. In developing this process, look for three things: (1) The opportunity to do something unique (and positive), (2) the opportunity to do something important, and (3) the opportunity to do something that resonates with the community. The third opportunity separates the healthcare profession from other professions.

The traditional notion that individuals are not true consumers of health services until they become sick has hampered the development of marketing in healthcare. Until recent years, no attempt was made to develop relationships with nonpatients. Prospective patients were not considered paying customers until they presented themselves for treatment. Progressive healthcare organizations realize that virtually all consumers are prospective customers virtually all of the time. They further realize that closing that one sale is less important than establishing a long-term relationship. The response, then, to the "when" question involves two answers: (1) all of the time; and (2) at every available opportunity.

THE FOUR PS OF MARKETING

In his book, *Basic Marketing: A Managerial Approach* (1960), E. Jerome McCarthy pioneered a set of variables that an organization can use to interact with its target market. The four components of the marketing mix—the four Ps—are product, place, price, and promotion. While these aspects of the marketing mix may not have the same meaning for health professionals as they do for marketers in other contexts, a basic understanding of them is necessary for an appreciation of the marketing process.

Product

The first P, the "product" of healthcare, represents the goods, services, and ideas offered by a healthcare organization. Ultimately, the foundation of marketing is a quality product, and a slick marketing campaign can never overcome a poorly delivered service. Today, the design of the product, its perceived attributes, and its packaging are all becoming more important for both healthcare providers and marketers.

Price

"Price," the second P, refers to the amount that is charged for a product, including fees, charges, premium contributions, deductibles, copayments, and other out-of-pocket costs of health services. In the past, price was not a differentiating factor—and thus not a marketing issue—among healthcare providers, but the emergence of managed care, elective procedures, and other phenomena is changing this. The issue of pricing for health services is a growing concern for marketers as developments in healthcare create price-sensitive customers in an increasingly consumer-driven environment.

Place

The third P, "place," represents the manner in which goods or services are distributed for use by consumers. Place might involve the location of a facility or the hours a health service can be accessed. As healthcare has become more consumer driven, the place variable has assumed a more critical role. In some cases, place factors may enhance perceptions of the quality of the product, as when a healthcare organization is conveniently located, facilitates access to care, or provides online services for more efficient service.

Promotion

"Promotion" is the fourth P of the marketing mix. Promotion refers to any means of informing the marketplace that the organization has developed a response to meet its needs. Promotion involves a range of tactics involving publicity, advertising, and personal selling. The promotional mix refers to the various communication techniques—such as advertising, personal selling, sales promotion, and public relations/product publicity—available to the marketer to achieve specific goals.

The organization's marketing mix ultimately reflects and determines its approach to the market. The role of the four Ps in market positioning, strategy development, and marketing planning will be discussed in later sections.

WE'RE NOT SELLING HAMBURGERS

Healthcare is different from other professions, and that's why most of us chose it. Health professionals, especially clinicians, fall into a special category, and the fact that clinicians—not administrators or businessmen—make most of the decisions with regard to patient care creates a dynamic unique to healthcare. Further, significant differences exist between healthcare consumers and the consumers of virtually any other good or service.

Healthcare organizations are usually multipurpose in nature, and large healthcare organizations like hospitals are likely to pursue a number of goals simultaneously. Indeed, the main goal of an academic medical center may not be the provision of patient care at all. It may be education, research, or community service, with direct patient care a secondary concern. Further, the not-for-profit orientation of most healthcare organizations and the frequent existence of government subsidies create an environment that is much different from that characterizing other industries.

Since we are not selling hamburgers, healthcare organizations involved in marketing establish a much different relationship with their target audiences than do organizations in other industries. For other types of products, a buyer-beware attitude exists. Healthcare consumers, however, are more willing to trust the messages disseminated by healthcare organizations. After all, healthcare providers are here to help us, not just make a buck. Echoing the doctor/patient relationship, the healthcare provider/healthcare consumer relationship involves a certain level of trust on the part of the customer.

The personal nature of health services involves an emotional component that is absent from other consumer transactions. The choices made by the patient or other decision makers are likely to be affected, as emotions like fear, pride, and vanity often come into play.

HOW DOES YOUR MARKETING EFFORT STACK UP?

A recent survey of 273 hospitals by the Society for Healthcare Strategy and Market Development (SHSMD 2005) found that in 2004 hospital marketing departments averaged 5.5 staff members and budgets of more than $1 million. Larger hospitals reported 10 or more staff members and budgets in excess of $3 million. The overwhelming majority of marketing executives were at the director or manager level of the organization, and nearly one-third of marketing managers held the title of vice president or senior vice president. Another SHSMD study of 706 marketing, communications, and strategy development staff reported in 2002 an average salary for marketing executives of $122,000 (SHSMD 2003). This compares favorably to the compensation of healthcare executives in other departments.

WHAT MARKETING IS NOT

We have discussed what marketing is, now let's discuss what marketing is not. Marketing is not just advertising, yet advertising is one key part of marketing. Marketing is not just PR, but PR is a vital component of marketing. The same is true for direct mail, telemarketing, sales, internal communication, and special events. Marketing is not embodied by any one technique, but they are all part of the marketing arsenal and should all be used within the context of the institution's marketing plan. All too often in healthcare the term "marketing" is used to reference one of these specific functions, masking the range of activities carried out under the banner of marketing and the extent to which marketing should pervade the organization.

Ultimately, no marketing silver bullets exist. Since no one is born a marketing professional, the healthcare marketer has to learn what works. Every organization is different, and you have to learn what works for yours. Since every market is also different, you have to learn what works in your market vis-à-vis the competition. And since every market is constantly changing, you must learn to be extremely adaptable. All of this underscores the point that marketing is a process used to manage your organization's reputation.

CREATING THE MARKETING ORGANIZATION

The challenges of marketing are easier to address if the organization is truly a "marketing organization." This means that the notion of marketing is incorporated into every aspect of the organization and that marketing principles guide decision making. The marketing implications of any activity should be considered, and all associates should see themselves as marketers for the organization. Associates are continuously quizzed on ways to provide better customer service, and corporate representatives keep their ears to the ground to identify challenges or opportunities arising from the environment.

An initial step toward becoming a marketing-conscious healthcare organization is including the appropriate personnel on the marketing team. While the marketing department or even an outside agency may have much of the responsibility for developing specific marketing campaigns, the overall marketing thrust should be driven by a core group of individuals representing administration, clinical operations, health information management, information technology, human resources, and research, in addition to marketing staff or consultants. Creating a team in this manner has the dual effect of ensuring an appropriate range of input into the marketing process and keeping all relevant parties informed of marketing strategies and promotional activities.

Businesses often find changing the institutional mind-set from sales- or operations-driven to customer-driven a difficult task. Healthcare in particular seems to have trouble making this leap.

HOW TO TELL IF YOUR ORGANIZATION IS A MARKETING ORGANIZATION

You can determine the extent to which your organization has incorporated marketing into its culture by the number of items below that apply to your organization:

_____ Do market data drive corporate decision making?

_____ Does a marketing executive sit at the table when strategic decisions are made?

_____ Do you know who your customers are and what they think?

_____ Do you know off the top of your head the strengths and weaknesses of your organization?

_____ Is there continuous two-way communication between corporate executives and the health professionals in the trenches?

_____ Do you have an overall strategy that drives marketing initiatives?

_____ Can you answer without thinking if quizzed about your organization's market positioning?

_____ Do you consider every employee to be part of the marketing team?

_____ Can all employees describe your organization's services?

_____ Do you maintain an in-house marketing team or have a contract with a professional marketer?

_____ Do you devote at least 2 percent of your annual budget to the marketing function?

_____ Are promotional activities by various subunits coordinated?

EIGHT MARKETING MISCONCEPTIONS

Although healthcare marketing has made significant strides as a profession in recent years, the industry continues to struggle with the appropriate role for marketing at the corporate level. As one hospital administrator put it: "Healthcare marketing is like a chameleon trying to walk on hot rocks. Not only must it dance, but it most constantly change its appearance."

In actuality the profession has matured greatly since the 1980s, becoming more of a science and less of an art, and finding ways to demonstrate its effectiveness to even its most vitriolic critics. Despite these advances, the full potential of marketing is often not reached because many in healthcare continue to harbor misconceptions about marketing. Some of these misconceptions are presented below, along with the actual facts.

Misconception 1: Marketing doesn't matter.

Fact: It may be better to say that marketing cannot change everything. Admittedly, there are some things that marketing cannot change but, even there, marketing can serve to explain, clarify and justify those situations. Effective marketing matters a lot.

Misconception 2: Marketing equals advertising.

Fact: All advertising is marketing but not all marketing is advertising. Marketing aligns strategy with goals and objectives, and establishes the framework for promotional activities. Advertising represents a tactic and a form of promotion among the many choices available to the marketer.

Misconception 3: Consumers rule in healthcare.

Fact: Consumers may be more important in healthcare today than in the past but, more often than not, they must be cultivated through indirect means. The best way to reach the consumer is through relationships with physicians, health plans, and other organizations serving the consumer. Consumers are becoming better at recognizing effective healthcare and are likely to respond accordingly.

Misconception 4: The size of the marketing budget determines success.

Fact: Big budgets make marketers happy but unless the money is spent effectively much of it may be wasted. Uniqueness in the marketplace combined with credibility and consistency are the three wise kings of healthcare marketing. Ultimately, how well the marketing budget is used is more important than its size.

Misconception 5: Public relations is not important.

Fact: Public relations is a fundamental component of the promotional mix. PR can take advantage of current events, timing, and marketing flexibility. The brand of an institution lives in the mind of consumers who evaluate your organization based on what they hear, believe, and remember. Public relations has the advantage of receiving third-party endorsement via the media.

Misconception 6: Clever names and logos sell healthcare.

Fact: Clever product names and logos might attract attention, but unless they are part of an overall package of services associated with the parent institution they may well compete with your institution's position in the market. The situation is analogous to a family reunion where the individuals are secondary to the family.

Misconception 7: Creativity drives the message.

Fact: People who judge marketing in terms of its creativity are typically not those consuming the services. Being creative for the sake of creativity only presents the illusion of marketing. Credibility, appropriate levels of reach and frequency, and competitive uniqueness have broader impact. If flashy marketing garners awards and not customers, the effort is wasted.

Misconception 8: Marketing fads generate new business.

Fact: While capitalizing on the current fad may be tempting, consistency really is king. The mind of the consumer is slower to hear than we are to speak. Their minds are even slower to believe what we say, and still slower to remember it. Using an "ad of the month" approach without establishing a consistent position for the institution is likely to result in a poor return on your marketing investment.

CRITICAL SUCCESS FACTORS

- Understand what marketing really involves and the various purposes it serves.
- Understand there are right and wrong reasons for marketing.
- Use marketing to shape and control your organization's reputation.
- Establish marketing as an ongoing, continuous activity.
- Integrate marketing as an activity comparable to other business functions.
- Establish your organization as a "marketing organization."
- Use marketing to inform and educate.

REFERENCES

McCarthy, E. J. 1960. *Basic Marketing: A Managerial Approach*. Burr Ridge, IL: McGraw-Hill.

Society for Healthcare Strategy and Market Development. 2003. *2002 Salary, Compensation, and Work Satisfaction Study*. Chicago: American Hospital Association.

Society for Healthcare Strategy and Market Development. 2005. *By the Numbers*. Chicago: American Hospital Association.

CHAPTER 2

The Marketing Process

WE'VE ALL HEARD the phase "fools rush in where angels fear to tread," and this is all too often the case with healthcare marketing. For years, most healthcare organizations resisted incorporating marketing into their corporate skill sets until they absolutely could not avoid it. Once they crossed the line, however, many began to spend marketing dollars like the proverbial drunken sailor. These impulsive reactions, usually in response to what the "other guy" was doing, reflected a failure to view marketing as a process. As a result, little real *marketing* was accomplished, but a lot of money was wasted on advertising, often to the detriment of the organization, its image, and its goals.

Marketing—regardless of the form it takes—is not a discrete activity but a process, and a much lengthier one than most healthcare administrators are likely to realize. Perhaps deceived by the facile presentation of advertising in the mass media, healthcare executives are often unaware that a clever 30-second advertisement is the culmination of months, if not years, of preparation. The end result of this process—a print or electronic ad, a telemarketing campaign, or a celebrity endorsement—represents a fraction of the total effort involved in designing, developing, and implementing the marketing activity.

Ideally, the marketing process should begin before the marketing campaign is ever formulated. The seeds of this campaign are found in two different components of the organization. First, the idea, approach, and methodology embodied in the marketing initiative should reflect the organization's strategic plan. That plan should in turn reflect the organization's mission statement, and the marketing effort should contribute to its strategic initiatives. If a marketing initiative cannot be traced back to its origins within the organization's strategic plan, serious questions should arise regarding why the marketing activity is being carried out.

The second component of any marketing campaign is located within the market research effort of the organization. While the odd situation may occur in which a marketing idea emerges spontaneously, the marketing campaign should originate from the groundwork laid by the research department. Marketing ideas should not arise *de novo* out of thin air but should reflect both the strategic orientation and previous market research of the organization. (All of this assumes, of course, that the organization has a strategic plan in place and ongoing market research capabilities, topics that are addressed in later chapters).

The steps in the marketing process are described in the sections that follow.

LAY THE GROUNDWORK

A need for marketing is seldom an emergency, although health professionals often approach it as if it were. As with most endeavors, do your homework; any marketer will require certain information before considering a promotional initiative. Information on the nature of the product offered, its differentiating attributes, and the packaging should be acquired. The extent to which other organizations offer the same service and the state of competition within the market area are important considerations as well. The marketer will want to know how the fee for the service was determined, what type of profit margin is anticipated, and how the price point compares to competitors' charges.

Service distribution information is required. Where are service outlets located? Can the service only be provided in a medical center location, or are there conveniently located sites for easy access by customers? The marketer must determine the extent to which the delivery of the service relies on other parties.

The overview developed in this manner represents the first step in the marketing process. Armed with this information, the marketer is in a position to begin formulating the marketing plan. At times, however, a marketer may indicate that the product is not ready for promotional activity.

STATE THE PROBLEM OR ISSUE

Defining the issue is a critical first step in the marketing process. Unless the issue is properly defined, the chances of developing a successful marketing campaign are low, so time spent initially isolating the issues represents a good investment. At this stage, the marketer is essentially asking, "what is the problem, why do we need to do something about it, and how can marketing be used to solve it? Is the problem that consumers don't know about our organization or service, or that they don't realize it is better than other options, or that they have negative perceptions that need to be addressed?" The framing of the problem will guide much of the subsequent process.

An example is used throughout this section to illustrate the marketing process. Consider a hypothetical freestanding diagnostic center that has recently acquired an "open" magnetic resonance imaging (MRI) machine that it wants to promote to the community. The marketing issue is, "what problem exists that this technology can address and how can our service solve it?" The follow-up question is, "how can marketing be used to facilitate this process?" The answers to these questions will serve as the foundation for the marketing initiative.

STATE ASSUMPTIONS

"Assumptions" are the shared understandings that drive the marketing process. If they are not specified early in the process, the marketing team may find itself well down the road holding conflicting notions of what the project is really about. The marketing team should agree on collective assumptions about the service to be provided and the target audience—its needs, preferences, and attitudes—as well as about the political environment, other options for services, the reimbursement climate, and so forth.

Some assumptions should be stated at the outset of the planning process. Others may develop as information is collected and more in-depth knowledge is gained concerning the target population, its healthcare needs, and the resources available to meet these needs. Assumptions will undoubtedly be refined during the marketing process; start by identifying general assumptions.

A marketer is not likely to be aware of all of the assumptions requiring consideration, given the complexity of healthcare, and in the rush to develop the marketing campaign, those close to the process may not devote appropriate attention to this step. The broad perspective of the administrator is critical at this point.

For the hypothetical example of the open MRI machine, make assumptions with regard to the demand for an alternative approach to conventional technology, the advantages of this technology, the willingness of the target population to adopt this technology, and the ability of the organization to capture patients from competitors who do not have this technology. Of course, assumptions regarding the reimbursement potential of such a cutting-edge technology are important as well.

REVIEW AVAILABLE DATA

The marketing process will invariably include a "discovery" stage during which the marketer determines what really is known about the situation. At this point the marketer can significantly build on the broad overview developed earlier. The information required is determined by the type of issue addressed in the marketing initiative. The kinds of information included at this stage are descriptions of

- the types of health problems that the organization, service, or technology can address;
- the size of the potential market;
- the characteristics of those affected by the identified problem;
- why a problem exists for certain patients; and
- why the organization's offering is a viable solution.

Note gaps in the available information and identify sources of additional information. Deficiencies in knowledge identified through this "first pass" of the data provide guidance for any additional research required later.

In some cases, primary research is required if the requisite information for developing a campaign is not otherwise available. This, of course, creates complications for the marketing process and requires additional tasks to be performed. A number of options are available for conducting primary research and numerous guides are available for consultation. More detail on this topic is provided in Chapter 3.

The information acquired through discovery is critical for justifying the marketing campaign. If any questions linger about the appropriateness of marketing as a solution for the problem, address them at this time. If the need for the service being offered cannot be justified, the anticipated volume is too low, the competition is too stiff, or any number of other factors exist, reexamine the marketing campaign.

Returning to the MRI example, identify how many people (suffering from what conditions) are in the market, what type of services they receive and from whom, their attitudes toward a new technology, their sources of reimbursement, and so forth.

SET THE GOAL

The goal represents the generalized accomplishments that the organization would like to achieve through the marketing initiative. The goal or goals established for the marketing plan should reflect the information generated by means of the background research and should align with the organization's mission statement and strategic plan.

The goal of the marketing initiative should be broad in scope and limited in detail. State the goal in a broad manner: "To establish Hospital X as the top-of-mind facility in this market area." For a service-specific initiative, the goal may read, "To dominate the niche for occupational medicine in this market area." There is a tendency to want to be much more specific, but save the specifics for the next step. The focus at this point is on a general goal.

In the case of the MRI initiative, the goal might be stated as follows: "To position XYZ Imaging as the premier if not the sole provider of alternative MRI capabilities within its market area." The specifics (e.g., what does "premier" mean) are not clarified here but are addressed in the next step.

DEFINE MARKETING OBJECTIVES

Objectives refer to the specific targets that must be reached to achieve the goal. While goals are general statements, objectives should be very specific and stated in clear and concise terms. Any concepts referenced in an objective must be clearly definable and measurable. Clear deadlines must also be established for the objectives. Finally, they must be amenable to evaluation. In the case of a marketing initiative, the objectives should be reasonable and reachable and clearly related to the ultimate goal.

Defining marketing objectives will help set priorities among possible promotional activities and determine the message and content requirements for each. Once marketing objectives are defined and reviewed by the appropriate parties, they serve as a kind of contract or agreement about the purpose of the marketing while indicating the desired outcomes.

A number of objectives are possible with regard to the goal for the MRI example:

- to raise the awareness of specialized services among consumers within the market area from a baseline of zero to 25 percent awareness within six months;
- to generate 100 inquiries concerning the MRI capabilities per month by the third month of operation;
- to stimulate a minimum of 20 referrals per month from other physicians by the third month of operation; or
- to increase utilization of the MRI equipment from a baseline of zero to an average of one scan per day by the end of the third month of operation.

FORMULATE A STRATEGY

Somewhere during this process, a decision must be made with regard to the strategy to implement. The strategy refers to the generalized approach to marketing best suited for achieving the stated goal. It should provide overall direction for the initiative, fit the available resources, minimize any potential resistance, resonate with the appropriate target audience, and, ultimately, frame the process for accomplishing the goals of the marketing initiative.

While the precise strategic approach may not be specified at this point, at least the options can be narrowed. This will serve to focus subsequent planning activities by eliminating strategies that are considered unproductive. For example, the target population may need to be educated on the issues prior to attempting behavioral change. In that case, the strategy would focus—initially at least—on education and information dissemination rather than "sales." In another case, initial research may indicate that a hard-to-reach population is not likely to be easily influenced by standard marketing approaches. In this case, a strategy involving partnerships with churches and other organizations in the community that reaches the target audience "where they live" might be necessary.

In the example of the MRI purchase, the unique nature of MRI technology may require more of an education approach than a hard-sell advertising approach. The assumption is that patients will gladly embrace the technology *if* they understand it, and that physicians will be willing to refer appropriate patients if *they* understand it. This approach might involve a series of infomercials, tours of the facility for office staff of referring physicians, and publicity through local news media.

CHOOSE A PROMOTIONAL TECHNIQUE

A number of options are available for promoting a particular service. However, the marketer must be able to discern the best method for the particular marketing campaign. The most effective approach is compatible with the intended audience's preferences, the type of information to be communicated, and ultimately, the goal of the initiative. Finally, the choice of promotional technique should reflect the strategy that has been chosen. The chosen technique should also consider a number of different factors including the context, the message conveyed and its tone, the timing of the promotional effort, and the channels best suited for disseminating the information.

Context and Message

The context refers to the physical and sociocultural environment in which the communication occurs. The message represents the information the marketer conveys to the target audience. Marketers must determine what information to provide, the presentation style and tone, and what the message must ultimately convey.

REALISTICALLY ASSESSING THE MARKETING APPROACH

Marketing is only one tool in the administrator's toolbox; in some cases marketing alone cannot achieve the desired goal. When addressing any business challenge, raise the question: "Is it really a marketing problem?" Marketing might not be the answer if the product is not perfected and/or appropriately packaged, if adequate support systems are not in place, or if the distribution channels are not well located. There may be no effective treatment for a particular illness, the target audience may be impossible to reach, or a solution may require currently unavailable services. It may be necessary to redirect efforts to these issues before attempting a marketing initiative.

In some cases, raising awareness or increasing knowledge among target audiences may be relatively easy. However, accomplishing such objectives may not necessarily lead to the behavior change requisite for reaching the marketing goal. Marketing per se cannot overcome product flaws, prohibitive costs, inappropriately located service outlets, or poor customer service. Indeed, the unforgivable sin of marketing is to begin promoting a product or service before it is ready for the market. Marketing is only effective if all of the other pieces are in place.

Timing

In marketing, timing is everything. In a mechanical sense, timing could refer to the day of the week or time of the day when a promotion occurs. It could also refer to the frequency of exposure established. Timing may also refer to the state of readiness on the part of the target audience vis-à-vis the message that is being conveyed.

Channels

Marketing communication uses a specific channel or channels, also referred to as the medium, and can involve interpersonal channels (e.g., physicians, friends, family members, counselors), group channels (e.g., brown bag lunches at work, classroom activities, church group discussions, neighborhood gatherings, and club meetings), or impersonal channels such as mass media.

In the case of the innovative MRI technology, consider the context, the message, the channel(s), and the timing of promotional activities. Given that the target audience for this service may differ from typical patients in some way, promoting this service in highly public group settings is probably not appropriate (although this might be entirely appropriate if the target audience is referring physicians). To the extent that the information can be conveyed to prospective customers in the privacy of their own homes via television or newspaper sources or, alternatively, through personal one-on-one consultation, the more acceptable the process will be.

The message in this case should be designed to clearly differentiate the new service and convey its benefits; it should be informative but in no way suggest that the overweight or claustrophobic individuals to which this service is targeted are considered inferior. The timing of promotions for such a service is tricky in that very few in the general population may currently need the service. The trick is to raise awareness of the service in the general public while at the same time making referral agents aware of its availability since they interact with patients at the time of need.

DEVELOP MATERIALS

Regardless of the promotional technique chosen, the materials required for a marketing effort require attention. Although message and materials development and production are often time-consuming and costly, these are critical steps in the development of a marketing initiative. Developing and pretesting messages and materials are important steps because they indicate early in the process which messages are most effective with the intended audiences. Positive results from pretesting can also generate early buy-in from others in the organization. Start with existing materials if possible, and determine what may be appropriate for the particular project rather than reinventing the wheel. Starting with this approach also contributes to the consistency of the image conveyed on the part of the organization.

Using the marketing strategy statement as a guide, take care to ensure that the message is accurate, current, complete, and relevant; that the content is appropriate for the intended audience; and that the materials are likely to meet the marketing objectives.

In the case of the open MRI, the primary need is for brochures designed for patients and physicians, respectively. Other materials needed include press releases related to this new service and materials documenting the benefits to health plans in support of reimbursement claims. To the extent that media advertising is used, advertising copy must be developed.

IMPLEMENT THE CAMPAIGN

Launching

Marketing staff must develop a launch plan for implementing the marketing initiative. This plan includes a schedule for preparing and distributing press releases, producing and distributing materials, planning and implementing tours and open houses, and preparing for any other tasks necessary to support the promotional effort.

The planning process creates a road map that the marketing staff uses to move the initiative to the desired goal. The campaign launch represents a transition from planning to implementation. Since the launch may involve various divisions within the organization, it is important to carefully coordinate the implementation. Given the need for cooperation among various parties within the organization, active participation by senior staff is essential.

In the case of the open MRI, the launch schedule must address the design and production of brochures and their distribution at sites likely to be visited by prospective customers, along with the distribution of a different version of the brochure to potential referring physicians and other referral agents. The schedule includes the preparation and distribution of press releases announcing the new service and the development in draft form (at least) of articles for local media. The launch schedule also includes the design and production of advertising pieces to be used in print media and a schedule for rolling out these advertisements.

Managing

The primary tasks involved in managing a marketing campaign include monitoring activities, staff, and budget; solving problems; evaluation; measuring audience response; and revising plans and operations as appropriate. The plan developed to manage the campaign should indicate how and when resources are needed, when specific events will occur, and at what points to assess the progress. During the development of the marketing plan, do not overlook the role of administrators in managing this process.

In regard to the MRI initiative, determine who will play what role and have what responsibility, how to coordinate the different components, how to manage the budget, and how and when to measure success. The overarching role of senior management in this process should be clearly specified.

Evaluating

The notion of evaluating the marketing initiative should be top of mind from the first day of the process, and the means for evaluation should be built into the marketing plan on the front end. This process should start in the early planning stages, at the time the goals and objectives are established.

Evaluation techniques focus on two types of analysis: process evaluation and outcome evaluation. The latter might be thought of in terms of short-term outcomes and long-term outcomes (impact). In addition, the financial dimension to the evaluation should be considered.

The type of process indicators used are determined by the type of initiative. In many cases, *operational* benchmarks are applicable to utilization levels, facility development, or staffing changes. *Clinical* standards are applicable to outcomes such as reducing the hospital mortality rate or improving surgical outcomes. *Financial* benchmarks are useful for such factors as revenue flow, profit margin, or return on investment.

Although evaluation techniques are often praised for their bottom-line objectivity, they are also useful in healthcare where it is not possible to place a dollar value on everything. Thus, cost-effectiveness analysis can take into consideration the intangible aspects of the service delivery process. (More detail on measuring the effectiveness of marketing is provided in Chapter 4.)

The evaluation process should consider the consequences of marketing activities—both intended and unintended. Indeed, early in the marketing planning process, when considering objectives, hypothesize about the likely consequences of the proposed action. Identifying the intended consequences is usually relatively easy; identifying the potential unintended consequences requires somewhat more creativity. The administrator should have ultimate responsibility for evaluation and is in a unique position to identify such potential adverse consequences.

In the case of the open MRI promotional campaign, the evaluation process should consider the extent to which milestones are being met (process) and the extent to which the general public becomes aware of the service, the target audience becomes familiar with the service, and referral agents are aware of the service (outcome). The number and place of articles and advertisements should be tracked.

The ultimate measure of effectiveness, of course, is reflected by the number of inquiries generated, the number of referrals made by other healthcare providers, the volume of procedures recorded, and the amount of revenue generated.

THE ADMINISTRATOR'S RESPONSIBILITY

In the past, the administrator's job was usually considered done when the marketing idea was turned over to the marketing department or an external marketing agency. Since a marketing campaign may be the primary exposure to your organization for much of the consumer population, such a hands-off approach is probably not a good idea. Indeed, in far too many cases the healthcare executive is shocked when she sees the deliverable in print or on the airwaves.

This is not meant to encourage micromanagement of the campaign on the part of the executive who doesn't have marketing skills. After all, marketing professionals often have an instinctual knack when it comes to producing a campaign. However, few generals will deploy their troops and then go about other business *assuming* that the war effort is on track. At a minimum some broad parameters should be of interest to the administrator: Is the approach in keeping with the strategic plan and our brand image? Can this really be done within the budget available? How are we going to measure the effectiveness of this campaign?

Marketers have a lot of different skills but they are not likely to have an overall appreciation of the organization, its goals, and its strategies. Someone with this critical perspective must remain involved with the marketing process. Executive oversight informed by a broad appreciation of the organization's position in the market is a critical contribution on the part of the healthcare administrator.

CRITICAL SUCCESS FACTORS

- Appreciate marketing as a well-thought-out, systematic process.
- View marketing as an extension of the organization's strategic plan.
- Use the organization's research as a basis for formulating marketing initiatives.
- Appreciate the assumptions that underlie any marketing endeavor.
- Know when to promote a product and when not to promote it.
- Involve senior management throughout the marketing process.

CHAPTER 3

Marketing Research and Planning

MARKETING RESEARCH AND marketing planning represent key components of the organization's marketing infrastructure. Marketing research encompasses the full range of research activities that support the marketing process. This doesn't mean just estimating the size of the market for health services but also involves research on the product, its pricing, its distribution channels, the nature of the competition, and any other factor that is likely to affect the organization's position in the market.

Marketing planning involves the development of a systematic approach to promote the organization. It can involve a short-term promotional project or it can be a component of a long-term strategic plan. It can focus alternatively on a product, service, program, or organization. Ultimately, the marketing plan formalizes the marketing process described in the previous chapter.

The twin pillars of research and planning provide the foundation for any marketing initiative. They represent the "heavy lifting" that lies behind a promotional initiative and account for the bulk of the effort that goes into marketing. Marketing research and marketing planning are important enough that they should be ongoing activities even in the absence of any formal marketing initiatives; they also require significant input from the administrative staff.

MARKETING RESEARCH

Any healthcare organization involved in marketing, program development, project evaluation, or strategic planning should undertake marketing research—that is, marketing research, like marketing itself, should be an inherent function of every healthcare organization. All organizations in healthcare today need to understand their market area, customers, and competition. The time when organizations could make decisions in an information vacuum is long past, and decision making must be data driven in today's healthcare environment.

When a healthcare organization misses an opportunity or makes a marketing mistake, a lack of research is often the culprit. Failure to conduct marketing research may result in a poorly located facility, a mistimed marketing initiative, a neglected key market niche, or misdirected product development. The costs involved in building and outfitting a clinic, developing a product, or mounting a marketing campaign are growing, leaving no margin for error in a competitive environment. It may require several good decisions for the organization to recover from the losses associated with one bad decision.

The historical tendency in healthcare has been to conduct research on an as-needed basis. "As-needed" usually arises when the organization experiences a downturn in admissions, shifts in referral patterns, a loss of key staff, or some other crisis. Because research activities do not directly produce revenue, an as-needed approach may be attractive to healthcare executives. However, the connection between marketing research and down-the-road revenue generation is very important, especially when new market opportunities are considered. While some research is admittedly better than none, research should drive the promotions rather than vice versa. "As needed" often translates into "too late."

Many healthcare organizations make the mistake of coming up with a promotional scheme before deciding to carry out the research. Conducting marketing research after a problem has already been identified is a reactive approach that places the cart before the horse. Research results are likely to arrive too late to be useful, and research that takes place after losses have been incurred and management is scrambling to "stop the bleeding" will probably be ineffective. Establish marketing research as an ongoing function that exists independent of any short-term marketing activities. Marketing research should drive the organization; the organization's marketing research should not be driven by the vagaries of the market.

Since the need for market intelligence is unpredictable, the organization should take a proactive approach to research. The time to start doing research is not after a competitor starts eroding your market share, a new service is suggested by the medical staff, a choice piece of property becomes available, or an unexpected niche emerges in the market. The healthcare organization should anticipate these developments and put itself in a proactive position. In the case of unanticipated developments, the organization should quickly and efficiently assess the situation and evaluate different options for action.

Effective marketing research is priceless to the organization because it can identify critical market trends and promising opportunities as well as quantify and measure activity over time. Marketing research can also help predict future consumer activity and anticipate consumer behavior. Such research can identify critical reasons why consumers make the choices they make, what factors they use to evaluate options, and which factors are most important to them. The regular feedback marketing research provides is important for tracking and measuring marketing efforts.

Ultimately, marketing research should drive both marketing and strategy development. Research should drive the formulation of any strategies, and the established strategy should influence the direction of marketing research. Since strategy development is—or at least should be—an ongoing activity, the marketing research function should be in place to support this effort.

Establishing a Research Function

Different organizations have different capacities for establishing a marketing research function. Obviously, larger organizations with more resources are in a better position to create in-house research capabilities or to engage marketing consultants. Being in a better position to do it, however, does not mean that the organization knows *how* to do it. Even hospitals that have established marketing research capabilities often limit the scope of these activities to targeted consumer research, marketing effectiveness evaluations, or customer satisfaction research.

Marketing research need not involve establishing a formal research department or allocating substantial funds. However, it does take a level of commitment on the part of the organization and someone with the responsibility for coordinating the research effort. The primary responsibility of management is to ensure that the appropriate resources are available and that an adequate research infrastructure is in place. Appropriate resources include internal or external marketing personnel and support staff, research personnel, data management capabilities (including geographic information systems), data resources (both internal and external), reporting capabilities, and evaluation resources.

Small healthcare organizations—which include most physician practices—may not feel that they are in a position to establish a research function. The typical healthcare organization, however, already has a head start on marketing research by virtue of the internal data at its fingertips (assuming it has effective IT systems in place). Routine internal data collected should indicate the types of conditions treated, the types of services performed or goods sold, the demographic characteristics of existing patients, the geographic areas from which patients are drawn, the payer mix of existing patients, and, hopefully, referral sources. By mining internal data, information can be compiled to support the marketing research effort.

The best option for both large and small organizations when it comes to external data is to identify a local resource already conducting similar research. Demographic analysis—an important starting point for any market research—is carried out by a wide range of analysts and, if local resources are not available, national firms can often provide this information. Universities are a great source of such information and often make the data available for free.

These same researchers or others may track business activity in the community. Since most healthcare organizations are considered businesses in this regard, community business activity information is likely found in their databases. Other researchers may specialize in health-related research and provide demand and utilization projections for various populations, specialties, or services. Since these analyses are performed on an ongoing basis, the costs are likely to be spread over a number of clients, resulting in a reasonably priced but highly valued product.

One option for external data is a "desktop" marketing system available from various vendors. Although considered pricy by many healthcare organizations, this option may be less expensive than gearing up the data collection and analysis process. Some data vendors offer online access to extensive databases, analytical resources, and mapping capabilities. Increases in the capabilities and user-friendliness of these systems make them worth considering.

Outside research consultants may serve as a useful adjunct to the resources available within a large healthcare organization, or as the main resource for a smaller organization. Outside consultants generally bring a broader perspective than that found within the organization, along with a degree of objectivity that may be compromised if the project is implemented using in-house staff. The outsider does not have to tailor findings to placate his manager and is generally free of the political considerations that inevitably arise within the organization.

On the downside, consultants may appear expensive and, at times, they are. Depending on the issues being researched, they may not have the in-depth understanding of the situation that an insider would have. And they may not be around when additional issues arise. Perhaps the most serious concern with outside consultants is the perceived threat they pose by raising issues that may reflect on the individual performance of the organization's staff.

One way to resolve the issue of whether to conduct research in-house or bring in a consultant is to ask some basic questions. Is it cheaper to outsource the work than to do it in-house? (This question assumes that the organization has a realistic understanding of the true costs of conducting research using in-house staff.) Does the research involve expertise that is not available in-house? Is special data, software, or equipment required, the purchase of which would not be practical for a one-time study? Is the issue at hand significantly controversial or sensitive as to demand the input of an objective outsider? Or, is the information of such a confidential nature that it needs to be kept "in the family"? Finally, the one question that should be asked with every proposed project is: Does in-house staff really have the available time and resources to conduct this project? Carrying out a comprehensive assessment of the true costs of the research effort is a prerequisite for answering these questions.

INFORMATION TECHNOLOGY AS A MARKETING TOOL

Marketing and information technology (IT) often have one thing in common in the eyes of healthcare administrators: They are both "necessary evils." Fortunately, progressive managers are beginning to realize that IT can actually serve as a marketing tool and thereby improve the efficiency of the marketing process and ultimately the organization's bottom line. IT is not an end in itself but supports the information management necessary for marketing research and marketing planning.

To the extent that the operations of the healthcare organization are automated, the information management system should provide the basis for the internal audit. The clinical management system and other internal systems can generate data on patient characteristics (including patient origin), health conditions treated, procedures performed, payer mix, referral sources, and other data required for an internal audit. Internal systems can also provide a wide range of financial data, including trends in revenue, revenue sources, collections, and other financial metrics.

To the extent that internal systems can interface with external data, these systems can profile the target population, identify opportunities for service expansion, profile competitors, calculate market share, and otherwise assess the organization's position within its market.

Given the importance of likely future developments for marketing planning, the information system provides the basis for establishing trend lines and projecting future levels of demand and utilization. Even if the internal systems cannot generate projections, the data they produce provide the basis for independent projection calculations.

More sophisticated organizations are capitalizing on their IT resources with database marketing and customer relationship management. For these organizations, data collected through operations, interactions with consumers, and marketing research create a platform that can be used for cross selling, up selling, repeat sales, and any number of other activities that contribute to increased volume and revenue.

The Role of Primary Research

Most of the research that has been described so far involves secondary data—data collected for one purpose but used for another (in this case, for marketing research). Many research questions, however, cannot be answered using secondary data. Unlike other industries, healthcare does not maintain industry-specific databases on which the researcher can draw. Even when national-level data are available (e.g., from the American Hospital Association), they are not likely to provide the level of specificity required at the local level. Thus, mission-critical data are often not available in healthcare. In these cases, primary research is clearly warranted.

Since the primary research process is expensive and time consuming, it should be the data collection method of last resort and should be executed only if certain criteria are met. First, the organization must have a clear vision of the purpose of the research, the questions that need answers, and how the findings will contribute to decision making. Second, data must be gathered in a methodologically acceptable fashion. This means that the organization must make a time-and-resources commitment to data collection and marshal adequate resources. Third, the organization must be committed to using the data, regardless of the outcome of the research. Primary research is of little value if an organization only accepts results consistent with the preconceived notions held by administrators.

A healthcare organization unaccustomed to carrying out market research is likely to face certain challenges in establishing this capability. Conducting primary research from scratch is difficult, and some outside resources will probably be required, possibly even to the point of fully outsourcing the research. Just as some national organizations will conduct patient satisfaction surveys, outside parties can be utilized for consumer research. In many cases, the possibility of piggybacking on an existing survey for a fraction of the cost of mounting an initiative de novo exists. In most cases, investing in existing capabilities rather than reinventing the wheel is the most efficient and effective approach.

Many healthcare organizations already have resources in place to support primary research. Larger organizations may be accustomed to conducting interviews with employees, and certainly every intake episode involves interviews with customers. Focus groups may have been conducted with employees, and this methodology can be extended to patients, referral physicians, and other stakeholders. If the organization is conducting patient satisfaction interviews, data collection resources may already be in place that can be shifted to other research areas.

MARKETING PLANNING

Despite all of the adages about the importance of planning, healthcare organizations often neglect this important function. Perhaps the most apt admonition is: If you don't care where you're going, you don't need a plan. Effective marketing planning begins with the mission and finds ways to enhance, expand, interpret, and execute it. Effective marketing planning is not done in isolation from the rest of the organization but contributes to organizational consistency, reliability, and responsiveness.

Marketing planning can take place at a variety of levels. At the highest level, a plan could be developed for a facility or a health system. A hospital that is attempting to "brand" itself might develop a master marketing plan to encompass virtually all aspects of the organization's marketing effort. Such a plan would be comprehensive in its approach and broad in its scope. Its time horizon may be relatively long in marketing terms (i.e., strategic), involving, perhaps, a two- to five-year planning period. At this level of planning, the administrator is likely to be most directly involved.

On the other hand, most marketing plans focus on a particular service, program, or event. A marketing plan developed to roll out a new service, office site, or piece of equipment, or a promotional plan for a series of patient education seminars, would be fairly narrow in scope and short-term in duration (i.e., tactical). The objectives would be more restrictive than those for a facility-wide plan, and different outcome measures would be applied.

As the steps in the marketing planning process are presented in the following sections, the emphasis is on the role of the administrator in this process.

Planning for Planning

The first step in the marketing planning process is "planning for planning." A basic understanding of the organization, its structure, and its functions should be developed at this point. A good starting point is a review of the organization's mission statement and any existing corporate goals. Much of the initial activity is organizational in nature and focuses on identifying the key stakeholders, decision makers, and resource persons that must be considered in the process, along with establishing a planning team to guide the process.

Stating Assumptions

Assumptions that will establish common understandings and provide the foundation for subsequent planning should be stated at the outset of the planning process. Assumptions may also be stated in regard to the nature of the market (and its population), the political climate, the position of other providers, and any other factors that might affect the planning process. Assumptions stated during the strategy development process are likely to relate to the organization's position within the market, the nature of competition, the distribution of the organization's facilities, and so forth.

Other assumptions will be developed as information is collected and more in-depth knowledge is gained concerning the market, its healthcare needs, and available services. While market analysts may be able to formulate assumptions related to tactical considerations, management involvement will likely be required for more strategic assumptions.

Gathering Information

The data collection process begins by gathering general background information on the organization through a review of any materials prepared about the organization and about the particular product or service to be marketed. This initial information-gathering process should also reveal something about the history of the organization, service, or product.

If a healthcare organization already has a marketing research function in place, it may be unnecessary to perform many of the tasks associated with initial information gathering. Typically, the marketing staff will have already examined most aspects of the environment as part of their ongoing marketing research activities and, at most, some updating of information on certain aspects of the environment will be necessary. In the case of a newly formed marketing department or the introduction of outside marketing resources, a wider range of data collection activities may be necessary.

Conducting the Internal Audit

An internal audit is useful in determining the nature of the organization and its marketing needs. Internal data can be accessed to develop an understanding of many aspects of the organization, including its products and services, the characteristics of its customers, and the manner in which customers are processed. Detailed information on existing marketing activities should be compiled. In performing the internal audit, the following aspects of the organization should be considered:

- services and products,
- customer characteristics,
- utilization patterns,
- marketing arrangements and resources,
- locations, and
- referral relationships.

The internal audit relies heavily on secondary data generated by the organization's data management systems. If adequate reporting capabilities are in place, compiling the necessary data should not represent a challenge. However, some primary research may be required to complete the internal audit. For example, computerized systems will not tell you much about patient processing, existing marketing efforts, or the customer service situation. Primary research techniques such as observation, interviews, and focus groups may be required to collect this information.

Conducting the External Audit

In conducting an external audit (or environmental assessment), broad social, economic, and political trends should be analyzed and their implications for the local environment considered. National trends in demographics, lifestyles, and attitudes should be considered for their impact on consumer behavior.

Trends affecting the healthcare industry should be analyzed as they relate to reimbursement patterns, changing organizational structures, the introduction of new treatment modalities, and so forth. The political environment should be assessed with attention to congressional mandates or Medicare policies at the national level, and to developments in certificate-of-need requirements and other regulations at the local level. Developments in the area of technology should be tracked, and advances in medical and surgical treatment modalities, pharmaceuticals, biomedical equipment, and information management should be monitored.

The analysis of the local market begins with delineating the market area and profiling the market area population. At a minimum, the analyst should examine the population in terms of age, sex, race/ethnicity, marital status/family structure, income, and education. The demographic analysis may be accompanied by an assessment of the psychographic characteristics of the market area population.

The health status of the market area population should be examined in terms of fertility characteristics, morbidity levels as indicated by measures of incidence and prevalence for various health conditions, and mortality patterns that reveal the relationship between death and the size, composition, and distribution of the population.

Health behavior involves both the formal use of health services and informal actions on the part of individuals designed to prevent health problems and maintain, enhance, or promote health. Indicators of formal health behavior include hospital admissions, patient days, average length of stay, use of other facilities besides hospitals, physician office visits, visits to nonphysician practitioners, and drug use. Informal indicators of health behavior would include information on lifestyles, prevention activities, dietary patterns, and risky behaviors.

The external audit should involve a competitive analysis that determines the position of the organization within the market. The degree of detail involved in the competitive analysis depends on the nature of the organization and the type of marketing being initiated.

Determining Strategies

The marketing planning process should always be guided by strategic considerations. The strategy chosen sets the tone for subsequent planning activities and establishes the parameters within which the marketer must operate. Ideally, the strategy employed for a marketing initiative will support the organization's mission statement and reflect the strategies embodied in the organization's strategic plan. The strategy could, for example, be framed in terms of an educational initiative, a public relations rather than an advertising approach, a soft-sell versus a hard-sell approach, and so forth, reflecting strategies established for the organization. (More information on strategy selection is provided in Chapter 5.)

Setting Goals

The goal represents the generalized accomplishments that the organization would like to achieve through the marketing plan. The goals established for the marketing plan should reflect the information generated by means of the background research and should be in keeping with the organization's mission statement. The goal of the marketing initiative should be guided by overarching strategic considerations rather than short-term tactical ones.

Setting Objectives

Having established a goal for the marketing initiative, the next step involves formulating objectives to support the attaining of that goal. Objectives should be clearly and concisely stated, and any concepts used must be easily definable and measurable. Objectives must be time bound, and clear deadlines must be established for accomplishing them. Objectives must also be amenable to evaluation since the success of the marketing effort is ultimately measured by the extent to which objectives have been achieved. Any barriers to accomplishing the stated objectives of the organization should be identified and assessed at this point.

Prioritizing Objectives

The objectives specified to support the marketing goal are likely to address different dimensions of the initiative. While all of the objectives may be considered important or even essential, pursuing all of them may not be feasible, at least not at the same time. Indeed, some objectives may potentially operate at cross purposes with others. The administrator should play a significant role in any decisions made with regard to prioritizing objectives.

Specifying Actions

The next step in the marketing planning process is specifying the actions to be carried out. It is one thing to indicate what should be done, it is another to specify *how* it should be done. A set of actions must be specified for each of the objectives identified. These actions take a wide range of forms, from ensuring that postage is available to support a direct-mail initiative to enlisting a celebrity spokesperson as a means of reaching an objective.

The action steps developed for a marketing plan may be relatively standardized. Marketing initiatives may already be under way, and some implementation efforts might already be in place. A reasonable understanding of marketing resource requirements is likely to have been previously established, and parties may already have responsibilities that could be shifted to the planning initiative.

Implementing the Marketing Plan

While the planning process has a number of useful purposes in its own right, the payoff comes in implementing the plan. The planning process creates a road map that the marketer can use to reach a goal. To approach plan implementation systematically, develop both a detailed project plan and an implementation matrix. The project plan systematically depicts the various steps in the planning process and specifies the sequence that should be followed. The project plan also indicates the relationships that exist between the various tasks and, more importantly, the extent to which completing some tasks is a prerequisite for accomplishing others. Managerial input is critical in developing the implementation plan given the need for resource allocation and coordination of effort.

The implementation matrix should list every action called for by the plan, breaking each action down into tasks if appropriate. For each action or task the responsible party should be identified, along with any secondary parties that should be involved in this activity. The matrix should indicate resource requirements (in terms of staff time, money, and other requirements). The start and end dates for each activity should be identified. Any prerequisites for accomplishing the task should be identified at the outset (and factored into the project plan). Finally, benchmarks should be established that allow the planning team to determine when an activity has been completed. The administrator is likely to have responsibility for monitoring the achievement of benchmarks.

Evaluating the Marketing Effort

Evaluating the marketing initiative should be top of mind on the first day of the process and, in fact, should be built into the process itself. It should involve ongoing process monitoring, including assessment of benchmarks and/or milestones along the way. Since the objectives of the marketing process are usually highly focused, measures of marketing effectiveness are both feasible and essential.

Evaluation techniques focus on two types of analysis—process (or formative) analysis and outcome (or summative) analysis. Both of these have a role to play in the project, although outcome evaluation is particularly important for the marketing planning process. Process evaluation should assess the efficiency of the marketing effort. For the outcome evaluation, changes in image or sales volume must be measured, and the success of the project must be calculated in relatively precise terms. Some form of cost-effectiveness assessment needs to be included. (Evaluation techniques are addressed in more detail in Chapter 4.)

A FINAL NOTE

When considering marketing research and marketing planning, the temporal dimension is very important. Collect data on past activities and current activities and, to the extent possible, include projections of future conditions. This past/present/future approach has relevance for the characteristics of the market area population and the organization's customers, the health status of the target population, health services demand and utilization, and other aspects of consumer behavior. While historical data provide a temporal perspective with regard to relevant trends, and current data provide a snapshot of the organization and its market at a point in time, the real value is in any projections of future conditions that can be generated.

Healthcare administrators tend to develop plans in response to today's situation rather than tomorrow's. Even when shown over and over that healthcare is a moving target, managers continue to act as if today's circumstances will persist into the future. This will virtually never be the case, so it behooves the healthcare administrator to be a champion for a future-oriented approach to research and planning. While the future is uncertain, being armed with an educated scenario of what the future will look like—and acting in anticipation of this future—is better than developing plans based on today's situation.

CRITICAL SUCCESS FACTORS

- Use marketing research to lay the groundwork for business development and marketing initiatives.
- Know where to obtain resources for marketing research.
- Capitalize on the organization's existing internal data.
- Develop a plan before attempting any promotional activity.
- Know how to prioritize marketing activities.
- Have a sense of the past, present, and future when developing marketing plans.

CHAPTER 4

The Dollars and Sense of Marketing

MANY HEALTHCARE ADMINISTRATORS still have a poor understanding of the financial side of marketing. This lack of understanding has contributed to the development of a love/hate relationship between the two. Hospitals in particular have been enamored with flashy (and expensive) advertising campaigns intended to capture the attention of healthcare consumers. They like the visibility generated by these campaigns, and some have garnered advertising and marketing industry awards. On the other hand, healthcare executives are not so enamored with marketing when they get the bill. Even administrators who haven't been involved in major marketing campaigns may have heard horror stories about big bucks spent on advertising—often with no apparent effect.

Such unpleasant experiences account for one of the major barriers to marketing in the minds of healthcare executives: the cost. In a cost-conscious environment, executives have concerns over the expense involved in implementing a marketing campaign, not to mention over the resources required for establishing a formal marketing program. The question that administrators ultimately have to answer is: How do we promote the organization without breaking the bank?

MARKETING AS AN INVESTMENT

Administrators have a tendency to perceive marketing as a necessary evil, a cost center that cannot be avoided in today's healthcare environment. This commonly held negative view reflects a misunderstanding of marketing and creates an artificial impediment to incorporating marketing into the organization. A more positive stance views marketing as an investment that, if properly made, will pay dividends not only today but also in the future. (Of course, this assumes the ability to measure the return on marketing investment, but more about that later.)

Like any investment, marketing involves a certain amount of risk (because the marketplace is constantly changing and shifting its priorities), faith (because fundamental rules exist that *should* ensure an acceptable return on the marketing investment), and trust (because marketing must be a team endeavor, a joint venture, and a collaborative effort within the organization).

Marketing should not be an expenditure made only for short-term gains, but an investment intended to reap future benefits. These long-term dividends extend beyond any direct contribution to the bottom line to the establishment of relationships with customers. At one time in healthcare the bulk of marketing was geared toward "making the sale," getting that customer in the door, or signing those customers up for an affinity program. Too much attention was paid to getting a $500 sale rather than obtaining a customer for life who would ultimately spend $250,000 on healthcare. The *real* goal of marketing should be to establish a relationship that will pay long-term dividends.

A useful example of marketing as relationship development is the patient satisfaction survey conducted after discharge. Ostensibly, the intent of the survey is to measure customer satisfaction for purposes of improving service in the future. But the simple process of collecting satisfaction data can be viewed as an opportunity for developing a relationship with the patient and the patient's family. Seeking input from customers and otherwise engaging them in dialog can serve multiple purposes. Seen in this light, the $15 that seems high for a completed satisfaction questionnaire doesn't look like much of an investment for solidifying a relationship with a potential lifelong customer.

On the topic of the long-term impact of marketing, don't forget the contribution that marketing makes to the strategic direction of the organization. How much is it worth to the organization to be able to identify a strategy that will result in increased productivity and profitability over time? The investment in the marketing research component by itself should pay handsome benefits to the organization by virtue of the guidance marketing provides for positioning the organization in the marketplace.

BREAKING THE COST BARRIER

A lack of firsthand experience with marketing means that many healthcare executives typically do not understand the costs associated with the marketing process. They may not appreciate the different cost components involved, nor the value of various marketing services. They may be aware, however, of the salaries of senior marketing professionals, the invoices for media advertising on which they sign off, or the sizable fees charged by an outside advertising agency. While these are certainly big-ticket items and part and parcel of the cost of marketing, they really don't reveal the true distribution of costs associated with the marketing efforts.

Indeed, to those unaccustomed to the marketing world, most quotes for marketing initiatives are likely to carry a certain amount of "sticker shock." Even healthcare organizations that generate significant revenue are generally not accustomed to the fees associated with some marketing initiatives. Concern over marketing expenses seems somewhat misplaced considering that, on average, hospitals spend well under 1 percent of their net revenue on marketing and communication activities. Viewing these expenditures within the proper context is important.

Two responses are generally offered when objections are raised to the costs involved in marketing. The first is the standard maxim: You get what you pay for. Cutting corners is always possible, but with most marketing campaigns you only have one opportunity to get it right. The cost differential between a good initiative and a great initiative is small, but the outcome gap may be substantial.

The second response is that marketing doesn't have to cost a lot. The organization is probably already involved in a number of relatively inexpensive marketing activities, and more formal marketing efforts can often be implemented without breaking the bank. Most marketing involves little or no cost—at least in terms of out-of-pocket expenses. An amazing amount of marketing can be built into routine corporate activities. Marketing can—and should—take place during new-employee orientation, customer service training, internal distribution of corporate materials, and so forth. Every regularly scheduled meeting can serve as a marketing opportunity.

MINIMIZING THE RISK, NOT THE COST

When a marketing issue comes up, an administrator is likely to raise the question as to how much should be spent. Whether to spend a little or a lot should not be the question. The real question is: What do you ultimately want to accomplish? Answer this basic question and the issue of expensive high-end marketing versus marketing on the cheap will be essentially answered. In answering this question, we need to consider short-term results, intermediate outcomes, and the long-term impact of the marketing initiative.

Ultimately, the issue raised by the healthcare executive should not be how to minimize the cost, the real question should relate to how to minimize the *risk* and maximize the opportunity. After all, the organization can always get more money but can it ever again benefit from a missed opportunity? One way to minimize risk is to seek out experienced, professional marketing personnel. Get the best talent you can and minimize the risk, not the salary. There is only going to be *one* grand opening for the new wing, *one* introduction of the new service, and *one* rollout of the organization's new brand. Quantifying the benefits of doing these right is difficult, but doing them wrong can result in significant fallout.

This doesn't mean, however, that every effort shouldn't be made to use marketing resources efficiently. "Overkill" is just as unproductive as cutting marketing corners. The trick is to determine the minimal amount of marketing firepower necessary to accomplish the marketing goal. Anything short of this is likely to reduce the effectiveness of the initiative. In a sense, the organization's marketing expenditures are insurance, and the downside of not having enough insurance is well known. Ensuring that risks are minimized should be the responsibility of the administrators involved in managing the marketing process.

TO MAKE OR BUY?

A decision that must often be made is whether to create marketing expertise inside the organization or use the services of an outside agency. Whether as simple as coming up with a name for a new service or as complex as developing a branding campaign, marketing professionals know how to do these things and know how to do them right. These skills are not likely to be found within the typical healthcare organization and are not easily or quickly developed.

Outsourcing Marketing

A number of options are available in terms of marketing arrangements, and each has different implications for the organization. One option is for the organization to fully outsource its marketing function. This approach was typical of many organizations in the early years of healthcare marketing and is still common among smaller organizations today. In this case, an entity or entities outside the organization handle virtually all of the activities related to the marketing process. The process can never be fully outsourced, of course, since the client organization must provide information on the product to be marketed, offer feedback on marketing strategies, and approve the materials that are developed. Most importantly, the administrator must be thoroughly involved in engaging and managing marketing resources.

Partial Outsourcing Under a Marketing Director

Another option for the healthcare organization is to outsource most of the marketing function, while carrying out some marketing activities in-house. This would typically happen in cases in which an organization has a marketing professional on staff but none of the other required capabilities. In this case, the marketing "director" coordinates the process but leaves most of the actual tasks to the agencies with which she contracts. In other cases, a large organization like a hospital may have some of the capabilities required for marketing in-house, but no formal marketing function. Its marketing staff may include copywriters, graphic artists, printing facilities, website developers, or other resources that could contribute to the marketing function. An outside marketing consultant may be required to glue all of these resources together.

In-House Marketing Department

A third option involves the in-house administration of most aspects of the marketing process. This includes establishing a formal marketing function with a budget, staff, facilities, and other necessary resources. This doesn't mean just hiring and turning everything over to a marketing professional, but it involves the full incorporation of the marketing function into the organizational structure. Even here, the organization is likely to continue outsourcing some aspects of the process, since the organization may not have certain specialized skills or the ability to perform certain functions. Even a well-developed marketing department within a healthcare organization is not likely to have the contacts and skills for negotiating media purchases or implementing a direct-mail campaign.

Some healthcare organizations are able to support virtually all of the functions required for marketing. Many multifacility health systems, for example, have a centralized marketing department. This department coordinates the marketing activities for the system and ensures that a consistent message is conveyed by all corporate entities. Even in these cases at least some functions may require outside resources, especially given the local character of both healthcare and marketing.

When considering outsourcing, don't be turned off by what appears to be a high hourly fee. These fees don't just cover an hour of labor, but pay for the years of experience and expertise behind that hour—and this could be considered priceless. If you have engaged the right marketing professional, that person will give you much more than an hour's work and may provide insights into a new service line or gaps in the market. While they are testing a slogan you want to use, they are probably also thinking about the next target audience to tap.

Obviously, the extent to which the marketing process is incorporated into the operations of the healthcare organization will determine the amount of control—and responsibility—the organization has over the marketing function. Even with completely outsourced marketing functions, time, energy, and money will be required of the client organization. If key staff have to spend two person-days, for example, explaining a complicated service to the marketers, considerable direct and indirect costs are involved. Diverting resources from other functions to the marketing campaign may involve unanticipated opportunity costs. Regardless of the option chosen, senior executives must continue to be actively involved. (Since a variety of options are available, any combination will be referred to as the "marketing resource" throughout the text.)

USE OF OUTSIDE AGENCIES

The Society for Healthcare Strategy and Market Development has released figures for 2004 on marketing activities for a sample of 273 hospitals nationwide. These figures are restricted to hospital expenditures and reflect actual practice rather than any ideal allocation of resources. Nevertheless, they provide a framework within which to view the outsourcing of marketing activities for any healthcare organization.

Activity	Percent Using Outside Agencies
Patient satisfaction tracking	81%
Collateral materials	77%
Advertising	76%
Marketing research	64%
Internet strategy/web development	50%
Strategic planning	34%
Marketing consulting	31%
Public relations	20%
Physician strategy development	18%
Event planning	17%

Source: Society for Healthcare Strategy and Market Development (2005).

PAYING FOR IMAGE

Decision makers may need to consider whether the marketing deliverable should be "pretty" or effective. While the general public (and some health professionals) may be easily impressed by slick-looking promotional materials, the administrator should step back and objectively assess the extent to which the materials contribute to the achievement of the desired results. Numerous creative and artistically crafted initiatives by healthcare organizations garner advertising awards but fail to accomplish the desired goal. Carefully think through any marketing initiative in terms of its potential impact. Assessing the aesthetic dimension and determining effectiveness are both necessary when testing a particular concept. Making a good impression is important, but closing the deal is the reason for the initiative.

The other side of the image coin involves the potential for negative consequences arising from a campaign. No one wants collateral damage from a marketing initiative and, as noted earlier, unintended consequences from such an endeavor are always possible. Even if consumers are not interested in the service, they will notice the look and feel of an advertisement. If the organization comes across as avaricious, uncaring, or insensitive, it may lose not only customers but also goodwill. Some marketers may not be aware of the nuances of healthcare delivery and inadvertently create campaigns that come across negatively. Oversight of senior management is essential in order to avoid this.

MARKETING COST COMPONENTS

The costs involved in establishing a marketing department are generally the same as for creating any other department. The components to be considered should address marketing research capabilities, marketing planning capabilities, marketing implementation, and marketing management capabilities. These could be represented by one person and some support staff, a team of marketing professionals, or some combination of internal and external resources. The costs considered should include both the direct and indirect costs involved. You should address these needs in the manner most appropriate for the organization.

Consider personnel costs (salary and benefits) along with any recruiting and training costs and standard overhead costs associated with operating the department and supporting the staff. Telecommunication and IT costs must be considered, as well as travel expenses and professional development costs (e.g., dues and subscriptions). The person who must pull the marketing plan together for the whole organization is the chief marketing officer, or whoever is assigned to serve this function, and this is one position for which you really do get what you pay for.

The costs associated with marketing research must also be factored into the equation, including both ongoing infrastructure expenses and nonrecurring expenses. These costs would include, in addition to the cost of research personnel, the costs associated with data acquisition and management, any out-of-pocket research expenses (e.g., for telephone surveys and market analyses), and any evaluation costs above and beyond core staffing.

Presumably, the marketing department will be involved in developing collateral materials (e.g., letterhead, business cards, and brochures), and the costs associated with designing and producing these materials should be factored into the budget. Any expenses associated with promotional items (e.g., key chains, pens, or refrigerator magnets) should also be considered. Also factor in the costs associated with exhibiting at trade shows.

Careful consideration should be given to the production of collateral materials. This is one area where executives may think with their egos rather than their marketing sense. Full-color brochures may be attractive and contribute in some way to furthering organizational goals, but given that they are likely to be distributed to employees or existing customers, they may constitute "preaching to the choir." They may also drain resources away from other marketing activities while failing to generate any new business.

Partly in response to the cost of collateral materials, a surge in "e-collateral" among healthcare providers has been noticed. Using the corporate website and other electronic means as marketing tools offers definite advantages over the traditional approach to collateral materials. This approach reduces the need for expensive print collateral while accommodating the preferences of consumers for easily accessed, customized materials.

With regard to a specific marketing campaign, budget items should address the cost for creative work, outside agency expenses, production costs for marketing materials, and direct mail expenses. Of course, a big-ticket item is likely to be media expenses. Television, radio, and newspaper advertising expenses often approximate the cost of operating the department. The importance of having an enterprise-wide marketing plan in place is obvious when the potential expense associated with media placement is considered.

An important consideration throughout this process is the non-monetary investment in marketing. These investments include the cost of intangibles that do not show up on the bottom line. At the top of this list should be the time and energy committed on the part of senior management. Senior management input involves time commitment and opportunity costs as managers are drawn away from other tasks.

Other indirect costs include the time and opportunity costs of managers of the services being marketed who may be required to spend time with the marketing staff as they develop the concept. Resources are likely to be required from the research, planning, or business development staff, as well as input from IT and health information management. Marketing input is typically not written into the job description for such positions, and time will have to be carved out from other activities, a realistic expectation if considering establishing an in-house marketing capability.

Marketing expenses should never be determined in a vacuum, but should be calculated within the operating limitations of the overall budget. Some markets are far more expensive to operate in than others. Some marketing activities are more expensive than others, some competitors are far bigger than others, and some medical specialties are more expensive to promote than others. The expertise of outside marketing professionals is likely to come in handy in determining these factors.

QUESTIONS TO ASK BEFORE SIGNING THE CHECK

In signing off on the budget for a marketing initiative, the healthcare administrator ought to ask several questions. These include:

- What do we really want to accomplish with this initiative?
- How does this effort relate to the organization's overall marketing plan and its strategic direction?
- Are other options available for accomplishing the same goals?
- Does this approach represent the best use of resources for accomplishing the desired ends?
- How well coordinated is this project with other marketing initiatives?
- Are there benchmarks that must be met before additional payment is remitted?
- Will we be able to measure the return on investment for this project?
- Are there any potential unintended consequences that may result from this project?
- Is this the best way to accomplish the identified objectives?

COST-EFFECTIVE MARKETING

Much of what falls under the heading of marketing does not have to be costly. A number of activities supportive of marketing can be carried out with minimal expense, some of them inherent aspects of the operation that involve little or no out-of-pocket expenditures. Certain promotional techniques are both inexpensive and effective.

The typical healthcare organization carries out many activities without any thought to their marketing significance. These include such diverse activities as using a state-of-the-art practice management system, establishing efficient admission and discharge procedures, generating bills that are easily understood, providing insurance submission guidance, and even maintaining an attractive and therapeutic physical plant. Although health professionals are becoming increasingly aware of the potential implications of functions that appear to be far removed from patient care, these activities are typically not carried out with marketing in mind. The trick is to tweak functions that are already performed to turn them into marketing assets.

Some activities that constitute marketing may not be obvious. These include such activities as communicating developments and new services to employees, providing a newsletter to patients and other customers, sponsoring a series of patient education programs, following up with patients after discharge, facilitating e-mail contact with providers, providing timely and thoughtful feedback to referring physicians, and conducting patient satisfaction surveys, among many other activities. These routine activities are generally considered part of the cost of doing business but are not considered from a marketing perspective.

A number of activities more directly considered under the marketing umbrella can be carried out inexpensively (more about this in Chapter 6). Many PR activities cost virtually nothing beyond the staff effort that is already being paid for. News items and articles in publications constitute free advertising and often require minimal effort. Visible participation by associates in community activities and the sponsorship of community events are low-cost activities that often generate considerable return. Public service announcements available to not-for-profit organizations involve only the cost of laying out the ad and can generate considerable response. Activities of the communication staff should all be considered marketing efforts. In-house publications should be the prime vehicle for internal marketing, and newsletters distributed to patients and potential patients should communicate useful information and lay the groundwork for future service utilization.

Even if paid advertising is deemed necessary, low-cost options can be considered. Banner ads inserted in newspapers and links on related websites are inexpensive and can generate significant exposure. Listings in the appropriate hospital or physician directories (usually free) can also be a source of referrals. Advantage should be taken of any opportunity for co-marketing.

COMPARATIVE MARKETING EXPENSE STATISTICS

The Society for Healthcare Strategy and Market Development has released figures for 2004 on marketing expenditures by a sample of 273 hospitals nationwide. These figures are restricted to hospital expenditures and reflect actual practice rather than any ideal allocation of resources. Nevertheless, they provide a framework within which to view the marketing expenditures for any healthcare organization.

Average marketing/ communication budget	$1,010,000
Percent of net hospital revenue	0.56%
Allocation by marketing function:	
Salaries	25%
Advertising	36%
Publications	10%
Collateral materials	8%
Community events/giveaways	8%
Marketing research	3%
Website management	3%
Call center expenses	2%
Other expenses	7%

Allocation of advertising expenses:

Newspapers/magazines	35%
Television	16%
Radio	14%
Yellow pages	10%
Direct mail	10%
Outdoor	9%
Internet	2%
Other	4%

Source: Society for Healthcare Strategy and Market Development (2005)

MAXIMIZING MARKETING BENEFITS

A key to squeezing the most benefit out of marketing efforts is to ensure that all such efforts serve multiple purposes. This is difficult to achieve with advertising which, by definition, has a very specific purpose. Even here, a print or electronic advertisement for a new service should additionally contribute to an enhanced image of the organization. Realistically, most consumers viewing the ad will not be immediate customers for the new service, but at some point they are likely to become customers for *some* hospital service. If the image conveyed is first class, the consumer is likely to remember that years from now.

One way to maximize benefits is through an integrated marketing approach. Integrated marketing or integrated marketing communication emphasizes the development of consistency within the promotional strategy of an organization. Integrated marketing communication encourages synergy between disparate activities to generate a more effective approach to marketing. Tighter marketing budgets have meant a squeeze on available resources, and the fragmentation of the media demands more coordination. The shift from mass marketing to target marketing and the rise of electronic media (especially the Internet) have contributed mightily to this development. In addition, many advantages to taking an integrated approach exist. Marketers are often able to coordinate advertising campaigns across varied media by supplementing, for example, television advertisements with marketing messages communicated via alternative media vehicles. Consumers may be exposed to print ads that capture a frame from a television spot, with a tagline that summarizes a 30-second commercial or a radio airing of dialog from the same TV spot.

Integrated marketing communication involves strategically choosing elements of marketing communication to effectively and economically influence transactions between an organization and its existing and potential customers, clients, and consumers; managing and controlling all marketing communication elements; and ensuring that the brand positioning, proposition, personality, and messages are delivered synergistically across every element of communication. Obviously, integrated marketing efforts must be implemented by the marketing staff, but this is an area that will clearly require the input of senior management.

An integrated marketing process should produce

1. strategies that reinforce each other,
2. messages that are consistent,
3. the synergy derived from integrated strategies,
4. cost savings,
5. a consistent creative approach, and
6. a sustainable competitive advantage.

MEASURING THE RETURN ON INVESTMENT FOR HEALTHCARE MARKETING

Determining return on investment (ROI) for marketing efforts is tough in any industry and a particular challenge in healthcare. For many in healthcare, there is a lack of knowledge—or, at best, confusion—concerning the concept of ROI. What marketing ROI is depends on the organization and, to a great extent, the sophistication of senior management. Factors that make ROI measurement a challenge in healthcare include the time delay in the appearance of marketing results and the fact that the use of health services is often not triggered by marketing. Further, many efforts toward marketing health services simply don't have a measurable return.

The key to measuring ROI is the ability to control for the variety of factors that are likely to influence the use of health services. Directly measuring the one-to-one impact of marketing on health services utilization is difficult because the healthcare consumer may take a highly convoluted path in getting to the service provider. Health professionals should think in terms of "global" ROI—that is, ROI for the total organization, such as awareness levels, preference levels, image ratings, market share, referral volumes and sources, and patient satisfaction.

A number of conditions must be in place to calculate marketing ROI. These include detailed financial accounting capabilities, the ability to easily access needed information, and an understanding of the costs involved in providing a service. They include the ability to generate data on operations and patient characteristics and report these data in a usable format. They include the need to account for the indirect impact of a marketing initiative, perhaps three or four layers removed from the target project. They also include the ability to obtain feedback from consumers, patients, employees, and other stakeholders. The most important prerequisite, however, is the ability to control for the variables in the equation being created. Determining the extent to which the marketing initiative contributed to the outcome identified is important. (Marketing ROI will be addressed in more detail in Chapter 8.)

Administrative attention to ROI is important, and senior staff must support this effort with appropriate resources. At the same time, an executive should not micromanage the process to reach some arbitrary goal for marketing ROI. The administrator's main responsibilities are to establish the context and perspective for measuring ROI and keep an eye on the long-term implications of the marketing initiative.

THE MARKETING ORGANIZATION REVISITED

The challenges of marketing are easier to address if the organization is truly a "marketing organization." Not only should it display a marketing mind-set, but it should also develop an appreciation of marketing resource requirements and commit to providing them. This means more than just having a marketing budget, of course; it means the full-fledged incorporation of the marketing function into the overall operation of the organization. To determine the extent to which a marketing organization is being established from the financial perspective, answer the following questions:

- Are marketing expenditures viewed as an investment or as a necessary cost of doing business?
- Have key staff been made available to contribute to the marketing effort?
- Has senior-level management been involved in marketing budget preparation and financial management?
- Can senior management recite statistics on marketing expenses (e.g., total budget or advertising expenses) off the top of their heads?
- Is the marketing budget calculated independently of other budgets or is it a residual category after all else is expensed?
- Does the organization devote at least 2 percent of its annual budget to marketing activities?
- Has the organization committed the resources necessary to support marketing (e.g., research capabilities and IT support)?

- Have adequate resources been devoted to marketing research?
- Has the organization identified and established relationships with external marketing resources?
- Has a matrix been developed to illustrate the cost-benefits of marketing?
- Have capabilities been put in place for measuring the effectiveness of marketing initiatives?
- Have capabilities been put in place for measuring the return on marketing investments?

CRITICAL SUCCESS FACTORS

- Develop a rational perspective on marketing expenditures.
- Be able to conceptualize marketing expenses as an investment.
- Minimize the risk, not the cost of marketing.
- Know what marketing activities to perform in house and what to outsource.
- Understand the components of marketing expenditures.
- Know how to get the most market impact for your marketing dollar.
- Maintain ongoing management involvement in marketing budgeting.

REFERENCES

Society for Healthcare Strategy and Market Development. 2005. *By the Numbers*. Chicago: American Hospital Association.

Market Positioning and Strategy Development

AN APPRECIATION OF two concepts—positioning and strategy development—is essential for effective marketing. "Positioning" refers to the way an organization or a product is perceived by the target audience relative to other similar products. "Strategy development" refers to the generalized approach taken to meet the challenges of the market. These are two areas in which the available marketing resource and senior management must definitely be on the same page.

MARKET POSITIONING

The Importance of Positioning

Just as people have different positions within the "pecking order" of a family, healthcare organizations have different "positions" within the pecking order of the marketplace. Whether defined in terms of reputation, brand, or some other dimension, the organization's position reflects the manner in which it is known within the community. In fact, an organization can occupy *two* positions—one determined by statistics and the other by perceptions. On the one hand, indicators of your position, such as market share, penetration rates, service-line dominance, and so forth, offer an objective picture of one's position. On the other hand, a position exists in the public's mind—the subjective position. The conventional wisdom vis-à-vis the organization's position might be at variance with its statistical position. One goal of marketing should be to establish the organization's position in the public's mind at a loftier height than the statistics show.

By definition, a market position is relative and only exists in relation to the other players in the market. Thus, the organization's reputation is viewed alongside the reputations of all similar organizations. The best position, of course, is unique, positive, and attractive to the target audience. This stance assumes that management knows what constitutes a positive position in the mind of consumers.

As with other attributes discussed previously, management should determine the organization's position in the market on its terms and not someone else's. If management does not strive to establish and manage the organization's position, the marketplace will establish one. Thus, a major objective of the marketing effort should be to proactively define the organization's position in its marketplace.

Determining the Market Position

Understanding the characteristics of the market for both positioning and strategy development purposes is important. This means understanding the target audience and the competition. The market must be assessed in terms of its demographic characteristics, health service needs, and utilization patterns. The competitive analysis assumes an understanding of the organizations that compete with yours. Once your research has identified and measured the competition, effective positioning tactics can be devised.

Determining the organization's objective position in the market requires an ability to access and analyze both internal and external data and, ultimately, interface the two. An experienced researcher can lay out the competitive situation the organization faces as well as measure the strengths of competitors. Grassroots research may be required to determine the subjective dimension of the organization's position. This may involve consumer surveys (including patient satisfaction research), focus groups, and in-depth interviews with community leaders, health professionals, policymakers, and the organization's employees.

The one thing that may be worse than not having a position is establishing an indefensible position. An inappropriately positioned organization, service, or facility will not contribute to organizational success—no matter what resources are invested. Duplicated positions (i.e., someone else already occupies the position in the market), unimportant positions (e.g., free hospital parking), and off-the-issue positions (e.g., "We Care") are usually more of a liability than an asset. Ultimately, the position chosen should be credible, unique, and easily remembered; should relate to the organization's mission; and should resonate with identified consumer preferences.

Positioning can occur at different levels within the organization, especially in the case of a large health system. While the positioning of all components of the organization should generally align, there may be reasons to differentially position subdivisions, service lines, or products. At the same time, different positioning may be in place for the various aspects of the marketing mix. Thus, one of the four Ps—product, price, place, and promotion—may be emphasized over the other three, or different services may be associated with different marketing positions. For example, fixed inpatient services may be positioned in terms of the product while the network of urgent care centers may be positioned in terms of place.

STRATEGY DEVELOPMENT

"Strategy" refers to the generalized approach to be taken in meeting the challenges of the market. Strategies set the tone for any marketing activities (tactics) and establish the parameters within which the marketer must operate. The strategy chosen will influence the nature of the marketing plan that is ultimately developed and should guide any subsequent marketing initiatives.

The strategic plan should serve as the primary mechanism for adapting to an ever-changing environment. The emphasis that it places on positioning underscores its central role in organizational development. Indeed, the nature of strategic planning equips the organization to adapt to the changing healthcare arena. Ultimately, a strategically oriented organization is one whose actions are aligned with the realities of the environment. The strategic mind-set adopted by the organization should ultimately spawn a marketing mind-set.

Ideally, strategies are carefully thought out and deliberately formulated as a result of strategic planning. However, the lack of an articulated strategy does not mean that no strategy exists. Acts of commission or omission ultimately serve to create a strategy, so the lack of a strategy could be considered a strategic approach in a technical sense. As a result, many healthcare organizations end up with de facto strategies that were not deliberately formulated. These may result from the lack of a formal strategic plan, a failure to link marketing to the strategic plan, or a failure to clearly articulate marketing strategies.

Before discussing various types of strategies, it may be worth reviewing the reasons for developing strategies. Any strategy developed should

- provide direction for the organization or program;
- focus the effort on one of many possible options;
- unify the organization's actions;
- differentiate the organization;
- customize the organization's promotions;
- marshall the organization's resources;
- support decision making within the organization; and
- provide a competitive edge for the organization.

Selecting Among Strategic Options

A number of factors must be considered in selecting a strategy, including the nature of the organization and its mission, the characteristics of the market (and, more specifically, the organization's customers), and the nature of the competition. Unfortunately, no standard list of strategies exists from which an organization can choose. Each situation is likely to be unique and call for creativity in strategy selection.

An examination of the *strengths, weaknesses, opportunities,* and *threats* (SWOT) that characterize the organization (or service or facility) and its environment is represented by a SWOT analysis, which should be carried out as part of the marketing planning process. A strength can be thought of as a particular skill or distinctive competence that the organization possesses that will aid it in achieving its stated objectives. A weakness refers to any deficiency or weak link that might hinder the achievement of specific objectives. An opportunity is any feature of the external environment that creates conditions advantageous to the organization in relation to its objectives. A threat is any environmental development with the potential for weakening the organization's market position.

Market-Oriented Strategy. The information gathered on the market and the competition, along with the results of the SWOT analysis, provides the foundation for strategy development. One approach to this might focus on the market and yield a market-oriented strategy. Examples of market-oriented strategies used in healthcare include

- *dominance strategy*, whereby the number one player in the market opts to focus on maintaining this position;
- *second-fiddle strategy*, in which the "runner up" in the market concedes its second-fiddle status and acts accordingly, adopting what might also be called a "market follower" strategy;

- *frontal attack strategy*, in which an organization decides to directly take on the market leader or major competitors;
- *niche strategy*, in which an organization concedes that it cannot successfully compete for the mainstream market, but instead concentrates on niche markets based on geography, population groups, or selected services; and
- *flanking strategy*, in which an organization outflanks the competition by entering new markets, cultivating new populations, or offering alternative products.

Marketing Mix Strategy. Another approach to selecting a strategy reflects the role of the marketing mix in setting strategic directions. The marketing mix is the set of controllable variables that the firm uses to influence the target market. The mix includes product, price, place, and promotion. As noted previously, the strategy could focus on any dimension of the four Ps or it could cut across all four of them.

Product-oriented strategies focus on a good (or product line) or service (or service line) of the organization. The strategy is built around the qualities of the product, and the marketing approach attempts to capitalize on those qualities. A product-oriented approach might focus on a *unique selling proposition* and relate to the ability of the organization to establish and communicate a distinct product benefit. Alternately, a positioning strategy might attempt to enhance the public's perception of your organization's place in the market. Positioning strategies can focus on different aspects of a product, such as product features, benefits, usage, or users, or even its relative merits vis-á-vis competitors.

Healthcare providers have seldom employed pricing strategies in the past. Despite this, growing numbers of providers compete on price, reflecting, among other factors, the growing importance of elective procedures. "Price" can be used as a basis for competition for services that are discretionary and typically paid for out of pocket. Most cosmetic surgery would fall into this category and, as competition has increased among ophthalmic surgeons, ophthalmologists performing laser eye surgery have begun to compete on the basis of price.

"Place" refers to the manner of distribution for a good or service, and in healthcare this typically refers to the location where services are rendered. As the focus of healthcare has shifted from the inpatient setting to the outpatient setting, healthcare providers have been forced to pay attention to the location of services. While hospitals are effectively immobile, outpatient services can be established potentially anywhere. Those who seek to compete with hospitals have taken advantage of their relative immobility and established facilities in proximity to target markets. This is also in response to a new generation of healthcare consumers that demands convenience of location and easy access to services.

The most visible type of strategy employed by healthcare organizations is likely to be one that relates to the promotion of the organization or its services. Over the past two decades much of the marketing effort on the part of healthcare providers has focused on advertising, direct mail, and other promotional strategies. The limitations on competition based on product, price, and place have encouraged healthcare providers to attempt to differentiate themselves through promotional strategies.

Promotional strategies should reflect the overriding strategic orientation of the organization. If, for example, a hospital adopts a niche strategy, its promotional efforts should be highly focused on a narrow range of services and/or a highly targeted population. On the other hand, a hospital pursuing a full-service strategy is likely to employ an approach that promotes the organization as the source of virtually any service.

Similarly, the promotional strategy should reflect the approach to the market that the organization has chosen. If the organization has adopted an aggressive, hard-sell approach to the market, the promotional strategy should reflect this. Conversely, if the organization has adopted a soft-sell approach, this would be reflected in initiatives meant to educate the market. An effective promotional strategy requires an understanding of the various media available and the ability to craft a message with appropriate content and tone.

PRODUCT LIFE CYCLE AND STRATEGY DEVELOPMENT

The stage in the product life cycle that characterizes an organization (or service) has important implications for strategy development.

1. *Introduction.* The first stage in the life cycle for a product is the introduction or market development stage. At this point, a new service is launched. Because the service is likely to be innovative, most of the marketing effort is directed toward creating awareness and cultivating early adopters in the market. At this stage, there are relatively few competitors, and the service is not standardized. Entry into the market is relatively easy because there are few established players.

2. *Growth.* The second stage in the life cycle is the growth phase. At this point, the service has become established and accepted by the market. Expansion is rapid as new customers are attracted and additional competitors enter the arena. The service becomes increasingly standardized, although enhancements may continue to contribute to product evolution.

3. *Maturity.* During the third stage, the service achieves maturity. At this point, most of the potential customers have been captured and growth begins to trail off. Because few new customers are available, competition for existing customers increases. Service features and pricing are highly standardized, and little differentiation remains between competitors. The number of competitors decreases as consolidation occurs among the various players in the market, and entering the market becomes increasingly difficult for new players.

When a service reaches maturity, a different strategic approach is required. Options for stretching the life of the service include modifying the service, modifying the market, and repositioning the service. At this stage, the organization attempts to squeeze whatever benefit it can from the existing service.

4. *Decline.* At the final stage in the life cycle, the service experiences decline. The number of customers decreases as consumers substitute new products or services. Typically, a "shake-out" occurs among industry players as the dominant competitors squeeze out the less entrenched, and other competitors adopt a different strategic direction. Competition among the remaining players for existing customers becomes even more heated. Because no innovations are being introduced and the customer base cannot be expanded, the remaining competitors see an increasing emphasis on reducing costs to maintain profitability.

The strategic approach should reflect the stage in the life cycle of the organization or service being marketed, and this will influence the packaging of goods and services, promotional techniques, approaches to competitors, and relationships with other organizations.

BRANDING AS A STRATEGY

An organization's products, services, and promotional messages are like the cattle in a herd being driven to market. You want every one of them wearing your brand. People will see the dust first, then hear the herd, and eventually see the individual cows, and you want consumers to recognize to whom each one belongs. The brand becomes the composite of all of the organization's messages as they are condensed and remembered in the mind of the consumer.

An effective brand name evokes positive associations for the organization. The brand image indicates what business the company is in, what benefit it provides, and why it is better than the competition. Therefore, the logic behind branding is simple: If consumers are more familiar with a company's brand, they are more likely to purchase the company's products.

A company's brand also has significant internal value. A strong corporate brand generates and sustains internal momentum. Employees have proven to be more committed to the brand's promise if it is understood and supported by every key player. The brand should be seen as part of a campaign to improve customer service. To maximize the effectiveness of the company's brand, the brand must be understood by all relevant audiences: consumers, prospects, business partners, the media, and employees.

Establishing a brand identity requires several steps. First, the organization must decide what to brand. This requires careful consideration of the services it offers, the people who provide the services, the competitors' services, and the population served. For example, should the multisite system be branded, or does it make more sense to focus on a specific service line? Second, the organization must define its brand message. This encompasses deciding what message the institution wants to communicate about the service they have decided to brand. What aspect of the organizations should the brand statement highlight? Finally, the brand must be communicated both internally and externally. Internal communication is important to ensure staff acceptance and staff enthusiasm, which are necessary for brand success. External communication can take place through various channels such as business documentation and advertising. The most important aspect, however, is that the overall message is clear, consistent, and continuous.

Today's healthcare environment demands that every organization establish a position in the market and develop a strategy for aggressively protecting and enhancing that position. The situation requires a proactive approach vis-à-vis the marketplace that reflects the organization's mission and is integrated into the strategic plan. Much of what follows in this book focuses on the resources for supporting these activities.

CRITICAL SUCCESS FACTORS

- Always know your organization's position in the market, and recognize the gap between that and the desired position.
- Don't let the market determine your organization's position.
- Adapt the marketing strategy to the organization and its marketing challenges.
- Know where you are in the product (or organization) life cycle.
- Effectively use branding as a strategy.

CHAPTER 6

The Promotional Toolbox

WHEN YOU PICKED up this book, you probably thought it was going to be about the information found in this chapter. As you no doubt realize by now, the actual implementation of the marketing initiative occurs well into the marketing process. We have finally reached the point where it makes sense to discuss the range of options available when launching a campaign as well as the factors that guide the choice of technique.

DETERMINING THE PROMOTIONAL MIX

A young boy was watching a carpenter work on a house and was very impressed with the heavy box full of tools. After a while the boy asked the carpenter, "Which is your favorite tool?" The carpenter answered, "It depends on the job," he said, "I like the one that gets the job done."

To the marketing newcomer, an overwhelming range of promotional "tools" may appear available. How, then, is one to determine which technique is appropriate for a particular situation?

Here, as elsewhere, consider the goal of the initiative and the strategy being pursued when making these decisions. Within this broad context, narrow down the options. Like the carpenter, the choice of promotional tools largely depends on the task at hand. Presented below are some of the criteria that a marketer may use in narrowing the choices.

Time Frame

A major consideration, of course, is the time frame involved. In marketing, as elsewhere, time is money. A short-term campaign focusing on a one-time event will require quickly deployed promotional techniques. A long-term effort, such as an enterprise marketing plan, will involve a range of techniques that can be implemented over a longer period of time. Within the context of the long-term marketing initiative, some short-term marketing techniques are likely to be implemented simultaneously with more long-term efforts.

The lead time for a marketing initiative is an important issue and, if appropriate research and planning capabilities are not in place, the organization may find itself up against a marketing deadline. The first rule, of course, is that *everything* takes longer than anticipated, and, as noted earlier, there is always more to marketing than meets the eye. Certain techniques can be employed expeditiously, while others, such as a television ad, may require up to six months of lead time. Techniques that do not necessarily require a long lead time include PR and communication projects where the framework is already in place. However, do not assume that the PR and communication folks are sitting on their hands waiting for something to do. In today's healthcare environment they are likely to be spread thin already and may not be able to respond as quickly as desired.

Cost

Intertwined with the time dimension is the money dimension. If ample funds are budgeted for the initiative, you can literally buy the time and space needed to build awareness fast. If the budget is small, achieving marketing results will take longer. For example, media advertising can produce results quickly but is very expensive. Public relations may be slower to show results but is relatively inexpensive. Keep in mind both short- and long-term goals and develop a mix of activities to maximize reach and frequency while ensuring that *some* promotional activities are taking place throughout the entire cycle. This hearkens back to the notion of an integrated marketing approach.

Organizational Reputation

Another consideration in selecting a promotional technique is the nature of the organization, a particularly ticklish issue in healthcare. There is something unseemly about an organization called "Sisters of Charity" running a glitzy, hard-sell television campaign. Even simply calling a press conference might seem pretentious for a not-for-profit organization. Aggressive marketing tactics may be a comfortable fit for the pharmaceutical industry, but they usually don't feel right for patient care organizations. The technique chosen should fit the organization doing the marketing and, more often than not, the techniques will involve PR, communication, community outreach, and educational programs (think infomercials) that reflect the character of the organization. The importance of reputation should be remembered throughout this process.

Audience

Another consideration is the nature of the audience likely to be addressed. The size and location of the audience you are trying to reach are important, as are its demographic characteristics. Media experts know how to target the audience based on age, gender, and other attributes. Indeed, the realization that women make most of the decisions with regard to healthcare revolutionized the approach to healthcare marketing. Big audiences call for a medium with broad reach, making network television, radio, and newspapers good media choices in these situations. Smaller target audiences require more focused media, such as magazines, newsletters, and cable television.

Product

Considering what is being promoted when selecting a marketing technique is also important. We must continually ask ourselves: "What are we selling?" What is the idea, service, or organization that we are promoting, and what promotional technique is compatible with it? If we are selling an organizational image, then frequent television and radio commercials may be in order. If we are promoting a new facility, perhaps PR, open houses, and sales calls to referral agents make sense. If an event is being promoted, we should probably focus on carefully placed print ads, public service announcements, flyers, and newsletter articles. Different products lend themselves to different promotional approaches, and some approaches are incompatible with certain services. A birthing center, for example, may call for a warm and fuzzy educational approach, the occupational medicine program may call for a partnership development strategy, and the cosmetic surgery clinic may call for a hard-hitting media campaign.

Message

The complexity of the message is another consideration in promotional decision making. A simple message like "Grand Opening!" is compatible with "big media," such as television and radio, but a complex message with a lot of details and specific responses is better for a newspaper-based campaign. If explaining a complex procedure to referral agents is necessary, the use of personal sales may be required. If you have a complex message in the newspaper you can always buy more space to talk about it, which is not an option in television and radio. The more specific the message is to the audience, the more specific your media choice should be. If you have a particular message going to a smaller audience, then direct mail, e-mail, or telemarketing can be very successful. The more specific the audience, the more direct your appeal to them can be.

Goal

The final consideration is the ultimate goal of the initiative. Do we want to raise awareness, change perceptions, convey information, or drive business to the organization? These diverse goals call for different techniques. Untold hours of research and considerable money are spent to get consumers to remember what the organization is. Even then customers do not remember verbatim what we said; they remember an abbreviated version of what was seen and understood. They create their own "interpretation" of our message (and generally what our message looked like). What they remember is a "lowest common denominator" of what we said. We must reach them with our message for them to be aware of it, and we must remind them frequently if we want them to remember it.

Don't forget the educational role of marketing—educating consumers, educating patients, educating staff, and educating policymakers. The ultimate defense for advertising or any other promotional technique is that it serves to educate the target audience. The frequent use of infomercials in healthcare reflects this emphasis on consumer education.

Ultimately, the goal of marketing is to drive business to the organization and away from competitors. Promotion is one way to accomplish this. Think carefully about which approach to feature and how to employ the chosen technique. Determine the best way to convince consumers to try our services (and not someone else's) and how to establish a long-term relationship. These objectives need to remain in the back of our minds as we consider promotional options.

Environment

One final point concerns the constantly changing promotional environment. Just a few years ago, no one would have predicted the impact of the Internet on the marketing arena. Changing consumer preferences, regulations that impact marketing (think about the Health Insurance Portability and Accountability Act [HIPAA]), technology developments, and other factors make the advertising arena a moving target. Media fragmentation has changed the playing field, and shifts in the media arena can be as important as shifts in healthcare. These developments include specialized media, such as community newspapers, cable television stations, specialized radio, health-related publications (the trade press), foreign-language publications or broadcast media, Internet "e-zines," and websites. These media may have a greater incentive to use a feature story or news item than general newspapers or regular television stations, and they can ensure an audience at a press conference even if the mainstream media don't show up.

Some media outlive their usefulness; others receive new life due to the changing environment. Discarded approaches to promotions can take on renewed importance as the healthcare environment evolves. Further, marketing is subject to fads just like every other field. The challenge is to be aware of the fads but not get caught up in mass hysteria—that is, to be contemporary but not trendy. The impetus for an initiative should originate with the strategic framework and the marketing plan, not from the current popularity of a promotional technique.

"HOOKING" THE CUSTOMER

Promotion within the healthcare marketplace is admittedly different from the promotional tactics used by Joe's Auto Parts. All

Joe has to do is get you to remember his name the next time you have car trouble. Nevertheless, the healthcare marketer, like Joe, has to find a way to "hook" prospective customers and keep them coming back. This is one of the greatest challenges in a competitive healthcare environment because the hooking process generally has to be much more subtle than in other industries. The trick is to convert existing activities of healthcare organizations into business magnets, whether this means attracting participants for a one-time event or establishing a lifelong relationship. Routine activities of healthcare organizations, such as health fairs, community education programs, and open houses, can be viewed as mechanisms to hook customers.

Promotion in healthcare is different because we are not just trying to make a sale—we are also trying to get the consumer to go to the right place at the right time to receive the right care. From the outset, promotional efforts should do more than just sell. They should educate, instruct, and direct consumers to the proper place for care, depending of course on the needs of each individual. In healthcare, relationships with consumers are based on customers getting exactly what they need the first time and in the most efficient manner possible. Consumers must believe we will live up to our end of the bargain in providing the most appropriate care. This educational element sets healthcare apart from other industries.

Transmitting all necessary knowledge about promotional techniques is impossible in the space available. The intent of this section is to raise awareness of the range of possibilities, indicate some of the trends in promotional options, and highlight some particularly relevant techniques.

CHOOSING A PROMOTIONAL TECHNIQUE

The selection of the promotional technique should always occur near the end of the process—that is, after every other marketing decision has been made. Far too often we jump ahead to media options and neglect marketing planning. A conversation with an administrator that begins with "I want you to come up with a newspaper ad that says..." usually means trouble. Why? Because it subverts the discipline instilled by following the marketing process and leapfrogs directly to the execution of the campaign. Every time this ready-fire-aim approach is employed it weakens the overall marketing plan.

Public Relations

Public relations is a form of promotion that uses publicity and other nonpaid forms of promotion and information dissemination in an attempt to influence feelings, opinions, or beliefs about the organization and its services. Public relations includes press releases, press conferences, distribution of feature stories to the media, public service announcements, and other publicity-oriented activities. Core functions include gathering media representatives for announcements and distributing news releases describing some newsworthy event or activity with the hope of getting press coverage. Effective PR is an art, so identifying an experienced professional who can mentor and train senior management and key staff in media relations is important.

Communication

Healthcare organizations typically establish mechanisms for communicating with their constituencies (both internal and external). Communication staff develop materials to disseminate to the public and to the employees of the organization. Internal newsletters and publications geared to relevant customer groups (e.g., patients, enrollees) are produced and patient education materials are frequently developed by communications staff. Separate communication departments may be established, or this function may overlap with the PR or community outreach functions. Effective communication is critical to the goal of educating the audience and crucial for the often-overlooked internal marketing effort. Even the most sophisticated marketing campaign will struggle without employee support.

Increased communication options, especially the Internet, have expanded the horizons for communication initiatives. In addition to publications geared to internal audiences or existing customers, options include publications in newspapers, newsletters, professional journals, and magazines, which have a seemingly insatiable hunger for health-related articles, columns, and how-to pieces.

Television and radio programming typically includes news programs, and healthcare continues to be a hot topic. Many health-related feature programs exist, and, indeed, entire networks are devoted to health-related topics. Television also offers the opportunity for dramatic programming, using investigative journalism and drama productions to highlight health-related issues. Radio offers some of the same opportunities for education-oriented programming.

The Internet has become the communication medium of choice for a growing number of healthcare consumers. The websites of healthcare organizations are increasingly designed to draw consumers and existing customers to the site and occupy them with a variety of information resources and interactive programs. The Internet supports the ability to transmit information in a variety of ways, including through informative websites, e-mails, chat rooms, and newsgroups.

Government Relations

Long before most healthcare organizations considered incorporating of a formal marketing function, they were involved in government relations activities. Healthcare organizations are typically regulated by agencies within their states, and for some purposes by federal agencies. The reimbursement available to healthcare providers may be controlled by these agencies, and not-for-profit organizations must continuously demonstrate to government agencies that they deserve their tax-exempt status. For these reasons, healthcare organizations must maintain discourse with a variety of government agencies, cultivate relationships with politicians and other policymakers, and often initiate lobbying activities directed toward various levels of government. This is one aspect of promotion that calls for direct involvement of both experienced professionals and senior management.

Community Outreach

Community outreach is a form of marketing that seeks to present the programs of the organization to the community and establish relationships with community organizations. Community outreach may involve episodic activities such as health fairs or educational programs for community residents. This function may also include ongoing initiatives involving outreach workers who are visible within the community on a recurring basis. This aspect of marketing emphasizes the organization's commitment to the community and its support of community organizations. While the benefits of community outreach activities are not as easily measured as some more direct marketing activities, the organization often gains customers as a result of its health screening activities, follow-up from educational seminars, or outreach worker referrals.

One objective of community outreach initiatives is to generate word-of-mouth (WOM) communication concerning the organization or its services. Word-of-mouth communication occurs when people share information about products or promotions with friends. Efforts to generate positive WOM support are important since WOM communication tends to be negative.

Networking

Networking involves developing and nurturing relationships with individuals and organizations with which mutually beneficial transactions might be carried out. As such, networking is probably the least formal of the various promotional techniques. Physicians and other clinicians, who until recently would never have agreed to advertise, actively network among their colleagues. A specialist may casually run into potential referring physicians at the country club or attend meetings that involve potential clients, partners, or referral agents. Arranging activities (e.g., golf tournaments) that would bring together various parties with whom one may want to interact would be another form of networking. Networking is particularly effective when dealing with parties with whom it is particularly difficult to get "face time" or when an informal setting involving personal interaction is required. Given the importance of relationship development at the highest levels of complementary organizations, such networking is an activity that should be carefully planned rather than implemented on the fly.

Personal Sales

Personal selling involves the oral presentation of information through a conversation with one or more prospective purchasers for the purpose of making a sale. Although the idea of "sales" seemed abhorrent to health professionals in the past, the rise of business-to-business marketing and a more retail orientation in healthcare have made this an increasingly important technique. The establishment of programs in the areas of occupational medicine, sports medicine, and fitness training has created the need for sales capabilities on the part of healthcare organizations.

The primary purposes of personal selling are to

- find prospects,
- convince prospects to buy the product, and
- keep existing customers satisfied.

Thus, the role of the salesperson involves more than merely selling; it includes communicating with customers in the wider sense and performing market research.

Sales Promotion

Sales promotion refers to any activity or material that acts as a direct inducement by offering added value or incentive to the product for resellers, salespersons, or consumers to achieve a specific sales and marketing objective. The sales promotion mix includes

- health fairs and trade shows;
- exhibits;
- demonstrations;
- contests and games;
- premiums and gifts;
- rebates;
- low-interest financing; and
- trade-in allowances.

Consumer sales promotion methods have less application to healthcare than to most other industries, although both pull and push incentives are used at various times within the industry. The giveaways that healthcare organizations distribute are included in this category. Participation in exhibits and conventions is common among healthcare organizations, and those entities operating on the retail side are more likely to employ sales promotion.

Direct Marketing

Direct marketing involves transmitting promotional materials directly to individuals and households using a variety of techniques.

Direct Mail. Direct mail is a means of promotion whereby selected customers are sent advertising material addressed specifically to them. This was traditionally done through the postal service, but more contemporary approaches use fax or e-mail transmission. Everyone is familiar with the junk mail that regularly turns up in the mailbox. This is now being joined by unsolicited faxes and spam e-mail messages. Direct mail has not historically been considered favorably by healthcare organizations because of its negative connotations. However, as healthcare has changed, direct mail has begun to receive increasing attention.

Telemarketing. Telemarketing is a form of direct marketing that has generated considerable backlash among consumers. Most people are familiar with outbound telemarketing in which individuals operating from a bank of telephone sets, often equipped with computer-assisted interviewing software, call individuals from a prospect list to offer a good or service. Inbound telemarketing is more benign in that it is a means of channeling incoming calls to a call center that can appropriately route customers to the desired site.

The widespread use of the Internet has made the World Wide Web an arena for direct marketing. Consumers can be drawn to websites through various means, and e-mail can be used to push marketing messages to both existing and potential online customers. The computerized aspect of the Internet allows for the easy customizing of messages for different individuals.

Advertising

Advertising refers to any paid form of nonpersonal presentation and promotion of an idea, organization, or product by an identifiable sponsor transmitted via mass media. Common forms of mass media include electronic forms, such as radio and television, and print forms, such as newspapers and magazines. These examples typically represent high-end forms of advertising and are relatively expensive. "Big media," such as radio and television, has a big price tag, and practitioners must be very careful not to devote too much of the marketing budget to a single ad campaign. In this situation, time really is money—their time (and space) is your money. Print media, the other major category, includes newspapers, magazines, directories (think the yellow pages), and other "paper" forms of promotions. A third but less significant category includes outdoor and display advertising. The following sections present important considerations with regard to media options.

Electronic Media. Electronic media are considered the more glamorous of the various promotional techniques. Radio represents the oldest of the electronic media and has the advantages of being able to target specific audiences, generate interaction through call-in shows, and provide a wide range of options in terms of timing. Further, radio advertising is a relatively good value compared to other types of advertising, and it certainly involves lower production costs than television advertising.

On the down side, reaching a targeted audience means reaching a smaller audience. Competition for choice air times may be stiff, making the best times expensive. Preserving information provided via the radio to refer to it later is often not practical for the listener. Radio is probably underutilized in healthcare today and may have untapped potential for healthcare organizations.

By the 1960s, television had become the medium of the day and, for many, represents the first choice for communicating one's message. Television offers similar opportunities to radio but with the advantage of video, special effects, color, and so forth. Television is driven by advertising and, with the advent of cable television, this medium represents an opportunity to focus on specific audiences.

Communication via television has the advantage of broad reach by means of network broadcasting or relatively narrow targeting in the form of cable stations. The viewing preferences of the intended audience can be exploited, and this may be an effective means of reaching low-income audiences who might not be accessible through other forms of communication. The production capabilities associated with television allow for high-impact, emotionally charged programming. Television involves high production costs for ads and high placement costs. It may not be possible to place ads at the most desirable time, and, more so than other media, television is characterized by communication "clutter," making it extremely difficult to attract attention to a particular promotional effort. The ability to retain information transmitted via television is limited, making the window for impacting the targeted audience relatively narrow.

Access to media has led to the growth of the infomercial as an acceptable method for promoting healthcare organizations and their services. Infomercials may involve a standard 30- to 60-second spot during which information is conveyed in an educational format, or even a 15- to 60-minute television commercial presented in a casual talk-show format that is designed to look like an ordinary television program.

The Internet is becoming the vehicle of choice for accessing health-related information, and this has two major implications for marketing. Paid advertising is found on many websites, and this area is expected to grow tremendously. Keyword ads displayed alongside search results remain the most lucrative format, accounting for as much as 40 percent of Internet ad revenues. The Internet has the advantage of providing information on demand and in whatever form the viewer wants to see it.

It may be worthwhile to insert a note on the vanishing public service announcement (PSA). In the past, not-for-profit organizations took advantage of free promotional space in both print and electronic media. Radio and television stations were required to provide a certain amount of free ad space for worthy causes in exchange for being allotted access to the airways, and media outlets did not mind using PSAs as filler when they had extra white space. As a result of changes in broadcasting regulations and the financial crunch faced by many print publications, the use of PSAs as a promotional tool is essentially a thing of the past. An opportunity to insert a notice in a publication may occasionally present itself, but this should not be considered a basic component of a marketing campaign.

Print Media. Newspapers are the most common print media, and communication in them can take a variety of forms. They offer a vehicle for paid advertisements and promotional inserts. Newspapers generally have broad coverage, can allot more space to a health-related topic than can electronic media, and, while the papers themselves have a limited shelf life, readers can excerpt articles about a health topic, notices of educational programs, and phone numbers of organizations promoting their services. Newspapers represent a "shotgun" approach to communication, and the organization has no significant control over who is exposed to the message. While the coverage is potentially very broad, readership of newspapers is steadily declining, they have lost some of their credibility a news source, and your message can easily get lost in the advertising clutter. Finally, newspaper advertising tends to be relatively pricy.

Magazines may not be the first promotional option that comes to mind for healthcare organizations, but this medium offers some advantages. Magazines are periodical publications that typically carry advertising. These include magazines aimed at the general public as well as trade publications geared to the interests of health professionals. Much business-to-business marketing takes place via trade journals and professional journals. Local general-purpose magazines (e.g., city magazines) offer opportunities for higher-end health services in that they generally attract a more upscale readership than newspapers. Such publications have the advantages of color production and a longer shelf life than newspapers.

Professional journals are possibly more ubiquitous in healthcare than in any other industry. Physicians and other health professionals are exposed to a wide range of journals. Every medical specialty and all allied health fields generate one or more journals. Major associations also publish regular journals. Some of these are academically oriented and typically do not carry advertisements. However, even mainstream medical journals like the *Journal of the American Medical Association* and the *New England Journal of Medicine* carry advertisements. These vehicles serve the purpose of "professional advertising" since they are geared to health professionals and not the general public. Pharmaceutical companies are heavy advertisers in these publications as are medical supply, equipment, and information technology vendors.

Directories have become an increasingly important means of gaining visibility for healthcare organizations. Some directories—such as state physician directories or the hospital association's hospital directory—are compiled for bureaucratic record-keeping purposes. These are not generally intended for commercial use, and an organization's inclusion may or may not be mandatory. Some directories are compiled for administrative purposes but are shared with a larger audience. The provider directory made available by a health plan or provider network includes only those practitioners that can be seen under that health plan.

Another category of directories are commercially produced for distribution. One function of these is to provide visibility to the organizations listed. There may be a fee for listing the organization, and the directories are typically sold to customers who need the information. Examples include directories of physicians, hospitals, information technology vendors, and so forth. A number of publishers compile and distribute directories as their primary business activity. An increasing number of directories are being posted on the Internet.

A commonly employed type of directory is the yellow pages. This traditional form of publicity has withstood the test of time better than some others and, indeed, hospitals still devote a not insignificant portion of their marketing budget to yellow pages listings.

One other print option is advertising inserts. These are enclosures used to relate information and are included as inserts in newspapers, magazines, and direct-mail packets. While ad inserts may not appear to convey the image a healthcare organization might desire, they do appear to be somewhat effective for organizations offering elective services (e.g., laser eye surgery) or more retail-oriented programs (e.g., fitness centers).

Display and Outdoor Advertising. Display advertising, including outdoor and transportation advertising, has become more common among healthcare organizations. Display advertising might include store displays, posters, and even bathroom advertising. Outdoor advertising includes billboards and advertisements on buses, taxis, and other vehicles (i.e., transit advertising). Display and outdoor advertising have the advantage of building awareness, wide exposure, relatively low costs, and flexibility in terms of frequency. Segmenting the target audiences is possible. Display and outdoor advertising in healthcare may have a certain negative connotation, although billboards remain popular as vehicles for healthcare advertising.

Posters are not likely to be the first promotional technique that comes to mind, but healthcare organizations may use them to promote an event or program. Posters provide instant visibility for a campaign and have the advantages of eye-catching design, the ability to communicate a brief message, and easy placement in key locations.

CREATING THE MEDIA PLAN

A critical part of any marketing effort is the media plan. Media planning involves matching the target audience to the appropriate media and considers the comparative costs of various media options. The plan includes recommendations on the combination of media that will be most effective in reaching the target audience and attaining the marketing objectives. Successful media planning requires the ability to identify, plan, and act on the best mix for the business. Any plan developed to coordinate the media effort should consider factors such as the nature of the local market, local cost variations in the various media, and so forth.

PUTTING IT ALL TOGETHER—REACH, FREQUENCY, AND CONSISTENCY

The best marketing efforts consider all of the choices and are carefully planned and laid out in advance so that promotional messages and media choices are combined to cover all important events during the entire calendar year. In other words, the marketing components should be well integrated. Integrated marketing or integrated marketing communication emphasizes the development of consistency within the promotional strategy of an organization. Its ultimate aim is to achieve synergy between component parts to generate a more effective approach to marketing.

To achieve this synergy, help will be needed from the advertising side. Someone with media-buying experience needs to be identified to help put the media plan together and obtain approval for it ahead of time. The person can be an employee, consultant, or someone with an advertising or PR agency, as long as they have the experience and the background to help you make good media and budget decisions. Eventually the organization's staff can learn this process by participating in it, but until then expert help will be required.

Remember, the best marketing initiatives can be described as "multipronged" and "integrated." Media that complement each other, address the various target audiences, and reflect consumer communication preferences contribute to the integration process and make for a more successful campaign. (Tables 6.1 and 6.2 illustrate the relevant aspects of various techniques.)

QUESTIONS TO ASK IN SELECTING A PROMOTIONAL TECHNIQUE

- Who is the target audience and what are its communication preferences?
- What is being promoted (i.e., an idea, an organization, a service)?
- What image of the organization do we want conveyed?
- What is the local climate with regard to various promotional options?
- What resources (financial and otherwise) can we apply to the initiative?
- How much can we afford to invest per unit of return (e.g., inquiry, office visit, procedure performed)?
- Will a given technique serve multiple purposes?
- Will a given technique be compatible with other marketing initiatives?
- What are the potential unintended consequences of using a particular technique?

And the most important question:
- Will this technique achieve the objectives established for the initiative?

TABLE 6.1—Matrix for Promotional Decision Making

Promotional Technique	Uses	Audience	Time Frame	Relative Cost	Advantages	Disadvantages
Public relations	Awareness Visibility Service rollout	General public Stakeholders Decision makers Influentials	Short-term within a longer-term strategic context	Primarily staff time with little out-of-pocket costs	Broad reach Low cost Short lead time	Not targeted Short shelf life
Communication	Awareness Visibility Education Relationship development/ maintenance	General public Stakeholders Existing customers Employees	Ongoing with periodic flurry of activity	Primarily staff time with moderate out-of-pocket costs	Direct to target Low cost	Narrow focus Staffing costs
Community outreach	Awareness Visibility Education Relationship development/ maintenance	General public Targeted consumer groups	Ongoing with periodic flurry of activity	Primarily staff time with moderate out-of-pocket costs	Ongoing presence Personalized Localized	High effort Long lead time

TABLE 6.1—Matrix for Promotional Decision Making (cont.)

Promotional Technique	Uses	Audience	Time Frame	Relative Cost	Advantages	Disadvantages
Networking	Awareness Business development Relationship development/ maintenance Intelligence gathering	Key stakeholders Potential partners Potential referrers	Ongoing	Little additional cost	Ongoing Targeted	Time commitment
Direct marketing	Exposure Product introduction Call to action	Targeted consumer groups	Short-term but with some lead time	Moderate cost Multiple exposures	Focused Customized Short shelf life	Low response rate High unit cost
Personal sales	Visibility Close contracts Relationship development/ maintenance	Influentials Potential customers	Regular, periodic contact	Moderate to high cost	Face-to-face Ongoing Feedback on market	Sales force maintenance Cost
Advertising	Awareness Visibility Image enhancement	General public Targeted consumer groups	Typically long term with long lead time	High cost	Many options Design options Easily targeted	Cost Negative connotation Short shelf life

TABLE 6.2—Matrix for Media Decision Making

Medium	Uses	Audience	Resource Requirements	Relative Cost	Advantages	Disadvantages
Television	Exposure Service introduction Call to action		Production skills Creative skills	High	Consumer appeal Multiple exposures	Cost Negative connotation Short shelf life Competing ads
Network		General public			Broad reach	Diffuse impact
Cable		Targeted consumers			Targeted reach	Narrow impact
Radio	Exposure Service introduction Call to action	General public Targeted consumers	Production skills Creative skills	Moderate	Broad or narrow reach	Cost Short shelf life
Newspapers	Exposure Service introduction Call to action	General public		Moderate	Broad reach Low unit cost Frequent exposure	Cost Competing ads Short shelf life
Magazines	Exposure Service introduction Call to action	General public (but higher end)		Moderate	Moderate shelf life Design options	Cost Competing ads
Internet	Education Channel business Relationship development/maintenance	General public Targeted consumers		Low	Appealing medium Interactive Ongoing	Incomplete coverage Spam annoyance

CRITICAL SUCCESS FACTORS

- Establish criteria for choosing among available marketing options.
- Ensure that all promotional activities contribute to the positive reputation of your organization.
- Know your customers well enough to employ effective promotional tools.
- Identify appropriate resources for developing a marketing plan.
- Use outside expertise as appropriate.

CHAPTER 7

The Changing Marketing Paradigm

THE HEALTHCARE ARENA is in a constant state of transition, and recent years have witnessed numerous developments with implications for marketing activities. Many of those trends remain in effect and new developments add to the turmoil within healthcare. The factors contributing to this changing environment must be understood to appreciate the marketing environment and to apply contemporary marketing techniques. Developments in the areas of healthcare, the marketing arena, and technology are all converging to create a new context for healthcare marketing. As a result, many believe healthcare marketing is not just changing but is being reinvented. Dynamic markets are constantly shifting and changing, requiring regular updates to the approach to marketing.

HEALTHCARE DEVELOPMENTS

Virtually every aspect of healthcare has undergone significant change over the past few years, and virtually all of these changes have implications for marketing. The sections that follow describe some of the major trends that are serving to transform the environment in which healthcare marketing is taking place.

Shifting Demand for Health Services

The demand for health services is influenced by numerous factors both inside and outside healthcare. Some of the emerging demand may be created by the industry as it introduces new products and services; some of it will be a result of changes in reimbursement patterns or the enactment of government regulations. Still more of the change in demand for services will reflect broad social trends that only have an indirect connection with healthcare. Regardless of the cause of the change, the nature of the demand for health services will be a major influence on future marketing activities.

Current demographic trends, for example, suggest an increase in the demand for gerontological services, women's services, and specialty care for baby boomers. We are already seeing a revival in the demand for inpatient care, and many facilities are scrambling to find space for their admissions. We can expect a decrease in the demand for obstetric and pediatric care but will likely experience an increase in the demand for gynecological services. Perhaps more than any other factor, the nature of the future demand for health services will influence the direction of healthcare marketing.

Growing Consumerism

Some observers have predicted that the first decade of the twenty-first century will be the decade of the consumer in healthcare, and ample evidence supports this assertion. "Consumer-driven healthcare" is one of the latest buzzwords in the field, and a "consumer choice" environment is emerging in which healthcare organizations will be required to cater to the needs and wants of a more demanding set of customers. These trends will require that marketers understand both the customer and the prospective customer better than at any time in the past, not only in terms of their demographics but also their lifestyles, attitudes, and preferences.

Increasing Competition

Healthcare organizations can expect continued competition for the healthcare consumer's business. Slow growth in demand, coupled with the continued entry of new players into the healthcare arena, is expected to raise competition to a level not experienced in the past. The monopolies that many healthcare organizations historically maintained have given way to cutthroat competition, and no component of the industry remains unaffected. Hospitals face competition from other hospitals, physicians (and other clinicians), and entrepreneurs who enter healthcare from other industries. Physicians face competition from other physicians, hospitals and urgent care facilities, and, increasingly, alternative therapists. Health plans face heated competition for customers, and the survival of managed care plans depends on their ability to successfully compete for enrollees. Even the pharmaceutical industry has become more competitive as the stakes have been raised.

The Dominance of Technology

Regardless of other trends developing in healthcare, the industry will continue to be technologically oriented. Even as some decry the impersonality of a technology-based system of care, the technological component is playing an increasing role in the provision of care and as a factor in the development of new products and services. The growing acceptance of electronic patient records and the eventual conversion of clinicians to computer enthusiasts will ensure that the industry is permeated with technology at all levels. These developments mean that healthcare marketers must be knowledgeable concerning the technology underlying the care they provide.

Traditional approaches to marketing are being supplanted by more complex methodologies that capitalize on contemporary technology. Healthcare marketers must incorporate a range of technology-based marketing techniques into their arsenals for use in cultivating the patient population. Techniques being adopted from other industries, such as database marketing and customer relationship management, must be understood and championed by healthcare marketers.

Increasing Costs

After a brief period of relatively moderate cost increases in the healthcare industry, costs are once again on the rise. The changing insurance environment and the emergence of a large elective surgery industry are making cost issues central to consumers, employers, and anyone else paying for health services. A lack of price-based competition and the extraordinary role of third-party payers have limited the involvement of healthcare marketers in the pricing component of the four Ps in the past, but that situation appears to be changing. Healthcare organizations are increasingly competing on the basis of price, and healthcare marketers must be in a position to support this marketing angle. Further, marketers are likely to be asked to explain to consumers why prices are increasing or how cost and quality of care may be related.

Focus on Outcomes

Driven by concerns over the effectiveness of the healthcare delivery system, persistent disclosures of medical errors in the system, and now the emergence of a pay-for-performance mind-set, healthcare providers are increasingly faced with the need to effectively assess outcomes. Marketers may be required to defend adverse mortality outcomes or, conversely, be presented with the opportunity to capitalize on favorable surgical outcomes. Marketers will be increasingly called on to moderate the outcomes issue, and outcome measures will become an inherent component of marketing evaluation. As a result, the marketer is likely to become the go-between for the provider and the public, regulators, and policy setters.

A Shift Toward Patient Management

In keeping with a broader definition of health and illness, the health-care industry is experiencing a shift away from disease management toward patient management. While no one is abandoning programs designed to manage the treatment of patients with chronic diseases, emphasis is growing on managing the whole person using a comprehensive therapeutic approach. This means expanding beyond the clinic's walls to meet patients "where they live." In effect, this becomes as much a marketing initiative as a clinical initiative. Tools of the marketer's trade, such as customer segmentation, communication, and social marketing, become essential for the shift toward patient management.

Growing Labor Force Concerns

Despite the weak labor market of the early twenty-first century, healthcare providers continue to face shortages of key personnel. The current shortfall is more extreme than previous ones, and little chance for short-term amelioration of the problem is recognized. The most highly publicized shortages are for nurses, but shortages exist for many other clinicians and technical staff, and now some are predicting a future physician shortage. As a result, much of the energy of marketers has shifted away from attracting consumers to attracting skilled personnel. Marketers must develop aggressive recruitment plans that help differentiate their providers from others competing for the same pool of workers. This is especially the case now that it has been conceded that salary is only one factor—and may not be the most important factor—that drives the decisions of would-be employees. Having recruited these key personnel, the marketer can then be expected to play a growing role in employee retention.

The Erosion of Trust

Perhaps the most significant development in the past decade in terms of effect on the healthcare-consuming public has been the erosion of trust in the healthcare system. Twenty years ago, physicians were accorded the status of demigods, and hospitals were held up as examples of efficient and altruistic institutions. Health plans were considered valuable safety nets, and pharmaceutical companies were hailed for their contributions to new therapies. Reports of unethical behavior, negligence, and greed have served to sully the reputations of most of the players in healthcare in one way or another. A spate of criminal and civil charges brought against healthcare executives have served to further create an environment of distrust and suspicion. As a result, a major role of the healthcare marketer in the future is likely to involve trust building, as efforts are made to repair the damage that healthcare has inflicted upon itself over the past two decades. Marketers will not only be promoting a product or service but also the image and integrity of the entire industry.

All of these developments have major implications for healthcare marketing. The future healthcare environment is likely to be characterized by more competition; tighter margins; more diverse, better-informed, and more demanding consumers; demands for accountability; and growing labor shortages. Marketing may not be a panacea for this laundry list of challenges, but the judicial use of marketing resources can certainly contribute to their amelioration.

MARKETING DEVELOPMENTS

The marketing field has undergone considerable transition over the past few years independent of its role in healthcare. This transition has involved more than the development of new promotional techniques or the exploitation of technology, but has also involved a paradigm shift within the marketing arena. These changes have affected everything from the look and feel of print advertisements to the philosophy underlying the marketing endeavor.

Shifting Perceptions

The tagline for this section might read: "The more things change, the more things change." No one ever had a successful marketing strategy that called for everything to remain just the way it was. While some institutions would like to retain a particularly advantageous position within their market forever, doing so is incredibly difficult and even then requires constant adjustments. This concept can be easily tested by jumping up in the air as high as possible. Two things invariably happen: You go up, and then you quickly come down. The marketing of a healthcare organization is similar. As long as you are active in the marketplace, your organization's awareness level will go up. When you decrease your activity in the marketplace, your awareness levels will begin to come back down. There is almost never a stable middle position. These constantly changing perceptions mean that marketers must be able to maintain continuous market presence. Even the market leader must respond and make tactical changes as events in the market occur and competitors shift their positions.

Shifting Delivery Channels

For marketing, the most significant changes involve the need to shift away from traditional channels (and marketing targets) to a much more diverse and dispersed target audience. For a pharmaceutical company, targeting 50,000 physicians in its specialty areas is significantly different from trying to reach 50 million potential consumers scattered across the country. While traditional pharmaceutical marketing approaches will not be abandoned, given this new emphasis, the drug company representative will be devalued in relation to the television ad agency. Additionally, a hospital schmoozing with the handful of plastic surgeons using its ambulatory surgery center has a significantly smaller potential impact than directly approaching thousands of potential cosmetic surgery patients. The variety of promotional channels has increased and diversified, with new options constantly being developed. Just a few years ago, who would have envisioned the impact of the Internet on the marketing endeavor?

Changing Audience Characteristics

Toward the end of the twentieth century, the American healthcare industry rediscovered the consumer. The consumer—the ultimate end user of health services and products—had long been written off as a marketing target. For most medical services, the physician made the decisions for the patient and, for the insured, the health plan controlled the choice of provider and range of services that could be obtained from that provider. Choice of drug typically depended on the physician's prescription, and supply channels in general focused on the middleman rather than the end users.

Today the effective marketer must be in closer touch with the end user than at any time in memory and must ultimately develop an in-depth understanding of the wants, needs, and preferences of the various categories of potential customers. The marketer must be able to determine who wants particular products and services and the extent to which a population category wants standardization versus customization. This will require marketers to develop an understanding of consumer characteristics and behaviors down to the household level, as is already being done in other industries.

Shifting Focus

The marketing field has undergone a significant shift in terms of focus over the past 20 years. The historical approach emphasized mass marketing initiatives in which a generalized message was transmitted to the public at large. The premise was that a homogenous market existed for a product and that a general, universal message was adequate. This was the state of marketing when healthcare organizations began to formally promote their services.

As more knowledge of consumers was generated, the emphasis shifted away from mass marketing to target marketing. "Target marketing" refers to marketing initiatives that focus on a market segment to which an organization desires to offer goods and services. While mass marketing involves a shotgun approach, target marketing is more of a rifle approach. Target markets in healthcare may be defined on the basis of geography, demographics, lifestyles, insurance coverage, usage rates, or other customer attributes.

As the targeting process became more refined, increasing interest was paid to micromarketing. "Micromarketing" is a form of target marketing in which companies tailor their marketing programs to the needs and wants of narrowly defined geographic, demographic, psychographic, or benefit segments. Customers and potential customers are identified at the household or individual level to promote goods and services directly to selected targets. Micromarketing is most effective when consumers with a narrow range of attributes must be reached.

Development of Relationship Marketing

Relationship marketing is the process of getting closer to the customer by developing a long-term relationship through careful attention to customer needs and service delivery. This stands in contrast to the historical emphasis on "making the sale." Relationship marketing is characterized by

- a focus on customer retention;
- an orientation toward product benefits rather than product features;
- a long-term view of the relationship;
- maximum emphasis on customer commitment and contact;
- development of ongoing relationships;
- multiple employee/customer contacts;
- an emphasis on key account relationship management; and
- an emphasis on trust.

All of the techniques discussed in the sections that follow incorporate at least some of these attributes. Ultimately, this approach represents a shift away from emphasis on a discrete episode of care toward the establishment of a relationship.

Perhaps the key message derived from these developments relates to changes in the manner in which organizations interface with their customers. The trends involve shifts away from impersonal one-size-fits-all marketing to personal customized approaches, from broad-based initiatives to narrowly targeted initiatives, from making the sale to establishing the relationship. The ultimate goal is to interface directly with the consumer in a manner that reflects that consumer's needs and makes use of the most effective means of communication for that consumer.

TECHNOLOGICAL DEVELOPMENTS

Nothing has offered as many opportunities to change approaches to the market as recent developments in technology. These developments have provided the ability to process unprecedented amounts of data at ever-increasing speeds. More importantly, these developments support the infrastructure necessary for the adoption of contemporary marketing techniques. Ultimately, developments in technology serve as catalysts for change and allow the opportunity to fine-tune efforts to build, nurture, and protect reputations. (The caveat to all of this, however, is that technology is a means of implementing a marketing strategy and not an end in its own right. Not having a marketing strategy is a good way to diminish the power of technology-based marketing techniques.)

Today, the availability of data has increased dramatically (although some notable gaps still exist), but the real advance has been in the ability to access, process, manipulate, and use data for marketing purposes. Information technology has emerged as an important force not only for operational aspects of healthcare but also for marketing. Once considered a necessary evil at best, progressive healthcare organizations have come to see the potential that IT offers. Far from being a liability, information management should be considered a valuable asset for the organization.

Information technology allows the organization to

- track trends and project them into the future;
- create "what-if" scenarios to test service offerings, pricing, and location options;
- identify patterns in utilization that can lead to the specification of opportunities (or threats);
- determine the organization's position within the market (especially vis-à-vis competitors); and
- identify opportunities that exist within the marketplace.

Of course, the ability to do these things assumes that the appropriate technology is in place, that staff are available to access the information, that the necessary skills are available for analysis and interpretation, *and* that top management appreciates the potential of marketing data. Any IT initiative should be carried out with this potential application in mind; if the requisite expertise is not available in-house, consultants can help acquire and interpret the data.

Emerging Marketing Techniques

As a result of the convergence of trends in healthcare, marketing, and technology, the healthcare marketing environment has changed and new promotional options have emerged. Virtually all of these innovations have occurred outside healthcare, but progressive healthcare organizations have begun adopting them for their use. The most noteworthy of these developments are described in the following sections.

Direct-to-Consumer Marketing. Direct-to-consumer (DTC) marketing involves promotional techniques aimed at the end user, targeted to specific customer segments, and customized to the greatest extent possible. The DTC movement is gaining momentum in healthcare as the industry becomes increasingly consumer driven and the ability to target narrow population segments is refined.

The trend toward DTC advertising is driven by a number of factors. Changed regulations within the pharmaceutical industry are a major contributor to this trend. The introduction of defined contributions that allow increased consumer latitude in choice of benefits has affected health plans, and managed care organizations are attempting to reposition themselves in the eyes of the consumer by offering customizable menus of services. Providers are increasingly chasing "discretionary" patient dollars (e.g., for laser eye surgery), and product vendors have discovered the Internet as a direct path to the hearts, minds, and pocketbooks of healthcare consumers. Healthcare marketers are modifying their methodologies to take into consideration the potential represented by 300 million prospective customers. This involves a radical rethinking of traditional approaches to the healthcare market.

Although the availability of the Internet has facilitated the ability to directly contact individual consumers, the DTC movement has affected other media as well. Television and print media have benefited from a considerable increase in expenditures, and direct mail appears to be making a comeback. While much of this has been driven by the pharmaceutical industry, it is reasonable to expect that other parties chasing these same consumers will follow suit.

This new environment is also likely to put the finishing touches on any one-size-fits-all approach in healthcare. The challenges for the marketer will increase by virtue of having to offer unbundled services to a wide array of potential customers with highly specific needs, rather than offering a bundled program to all customers. Take for example the health plan that has historically offered a "standard" package of benefits to all enrollees. With the move to a defined contributions approach, the marketer must be able to promote a variety of unbundled services to a variety of consumers with different needs and preferences. In the past, Employer A (with a blue-collar workforce) offered the same benefits as Employer B (with a highly educated, professional workforce). In the future, the plan being offered to Employer A must reflect the needs of the employees of Employer A and, of necessity, be different from the plan being sold to Employer B.

Database Marketing. Database marketing involves the collection, storage, analysis, and use of information regarding customers and their past purchase behaviors to guide future marketing decisions. In many ways, it epitomizes the interface of the various dimensions of marketing—the who, where, when, and what. It involves building a comprehensive database of customer profiles and initiating direct marketing based on these profiles.

Although database marketing is a well-established component of marketing in virtually every other industry, health professionals have been slow to adopt this methodology. The failure of healthcare to take advantage of data-oriented approaches has limited practitioners' competitive potential. Today, however, technological advances make it easier than ever to take advantage of these techniques.

Any choice-driven program is a natural for database marketing. This could include anything from affinity programs (e.g., seniors programs) for hospitals, to interaction with patients for physician practices, to fund-raising initiatives for healthcare organizations. Pharmaceutical companies are already using a version of database marketing to target customers in their DTC campaigns. Health plans are also beginning to use this approach for segmenting their enrollee populations.

In other industries, database marketing is used for cross selling, up selling, follow-up sales, and other activities that contribute to improved volume and revenue. Healthcare organizations are starting to expand their boundaries and think a little more broadly about the application of database marketing.

Customer Relationship Marketing. Database marketing is closely linked to customer relationship marketing (CRM). Customer relationship marketing involves creating a centralized body of knowledge that integrates internal customer data with external market data. This integrated data set can be analyzed to determine patterns relevant to an understanding of the market and its needs. This knowledge can be converted into a communication vehicle that allows the healthcare organization to target relevant prospects and deliver the appropriate message.

When CRM appeared on the health scene during the 1990s, few health professionals recognized its potential. However, more progressive marketers adopted the CRM techniques to aggregate all patient and market data into a centralized database. The goal was to gain more market share, and CRM, unlike advertising or other mass marketing techniques, allowed marketers to personalize direct mail and track campaign results. Today, health professionals have come to realize the extent to which CRM can serve to reinvent marketing.

Customer relationship management strategies may prove to be the next big thing in healthcare marketing, and for good reason. Well-thought-out and well-executed CRM programs are generating substantial returns for many businesses, and new technologies only add to the possibilities. Healthcare organizations are beginning to recognize the benefits of CRM, and increased spending on CRM activities is predicted.

The most important aspects of a true CRM initiative lie in how the organization as a whole defines its customers, identifies and segments their needs, and organizes around serving them in the most efficient and effective manner possible. Marketers should first identify what goals are most important to the organization, and these should guide the internal planning and implementation efforts. Some of the more common goals and objectives for developing and implementing technology-driven customer relationship programs include

- improving customer service and satisfaction;
- increasing profitability;
- reducing the number of negative customer experiences;
- allocating resources more efficiently;
- reducing the cost of managing customer interactions;
- attracting and retaining customers and prospects;
- staying in front of customers and building stronger relationships over time; and
- improving clinical outcomes.

Internet Marketing. The Internet has radically transformed the worlds of marketing and healthcare. Although healthcare organizations were slow to jump on the Internet marketing bandwagon, recent years have seen a surge of interest in the use of the Internet for a wide range of marketing activities. Almost all hospitals have websites today, and for many this has become their primary interface with their customers.

Significant growth has occurred in the number of consumers who search for healthcare information online. The Internet is used as a resource both before and after visiting the doctor, by both patient and caregiver. Public interest in online healthcare information continues to grow, and increasing numbers of healthcare consumers are logging on.

Healthcare websites have generally moved beyond static marketing information and corporate descriptions and have introduced a deeper level of service information, health content, and interactive features. Most, however, are not truly integrated with their other marketing efforts or other IT applications in the hospital. A small number of health systems are pushing customized health information and medical records out to consumers, allowing e-mail communication with physicians, and performing actual disease management online.

Healthcare marketers are successfully using offline techniques to draw consumers into their sites to search for information or respond to specific offers, such as finding a physician, viewing an infant photo, or signing up for a health screening. Once consumers are online, healthcare organizations are converting these "browsers" into prospects by capturing personal information in a customer database or having them sign up for interactive health news and medical reminders. This allows the hospital to continue marketing to these consumers in a more personal way than just advertising on television or through direct mail.

The Internet also has the advantages of being instantly updated and providing live audio and video feeds in the same manner as radio and television. Information can be customized for specific recipients, and the content can be carefully controlled. Further, the Internet offers the opportunity for interaction (think online health-risk appraisals) and the two-way transfer of information provides an advantage over other forms of communication. Unlike any other medium, the Internet serves as a window to an unlimited number of other sources of information.

THE WEBSITE AS A MARKETING TOOL: KEY SUCCESS FACTORS

Experience with using websites as marketing tools has taught us some important lessons. These lessons are distilled in the key success factors listed here. Note that little mention is made of the *technical* aspects of website development. This reflects the crucial role of nontechnical factors in the establishment of a successful site. Key success factors include

- a well-thought-out plan for developing the website;
- an adequate understanding of customer wants and needs;
- qualified professionals for design and implementation;
- careful consideration of website content;
- integration with other marketing efforts;
- realization that the project is never finished;
- a formal, long-term commitment on the part of the organization; and
- senior management participation in all aspects of website development and operation.

LIMITATIONS TO CONTEMPORARY MARKETING TECHNIQUES

The various contemporary approaches to marketing presented in this chapter clearly have useful applications in healthcare. Indeed, healthcare may need many of these methods more than other industries. However, barriers to incorporating some of the more innovative and technology-based techniques into healthcare exist.

Healthcare organizations often do not have the personnel or technical resources to implement the most complex techniques. They may lack the IT infrastructure and often cannot access data in the manner necessary to support some of these techniques. They are not likely to have the know-how to implement database marketing or CRM without bringing in outside consultants.

When it comes to data, not only do healthcare organizations often lack necessary data, but they also have additional concerns about the confidentiality of the patient data used. The enactment of HIPAA legislation has made many healthcare organizations gun-shy even when it comes to legitimate uses of personal health data. The conservative nature of health professionals presents a barrier to using data in ways that individuals in other industries would take for granted. As we have seen with the halting advance of healthcare IT overall, organizational and conceptual issues present a more significant barrier than technological capabilities.

A REMINDER

In light of the frequent developments in healthcare, technology, and marketing techniques, the implementation of marketing activities might divert the marketer from the established mission, strategy, and plan. Successful marketing demands the discipline required to make this linkage. No matter how glamorous marketing tactics may be, their roots must be firmly planted within the marketing plan, consciously reflect that plan, and ultimately be traceable back to the organization's mission. Making these links is always a challenge for healthcare marketers, and the turbulence of the marketing environment makes the task even more of a challenge. The ability to make this connection, however, is likely to be the key factor in long-term marketing success or failure.

CRITICAL SUCCESS FACTORS

- Keep abreast of changes in the healthcare environment.
- Use marketing as a tool for adapting to a changing environment.
- Establish an adequate information management infrastructure.
- Perceive information management as a marketing support system.
- Capitalize on technology-based marketing techniques.
- Be aware of the limitations of marketing technology in healthcare.
- Develop a website that drives business to your organization.

CHAPTER 8

Measuring the Effectiveness of Marketing

EVALUATING THE EFFECTIVENESS of a marketing initiative is often an afterthought—and this is particularly the case in healthcare. Failing to measure the impact of marketing initiatives limits the ability of healthcare organizations to justify the costs involved in the effort. Since marketers are likely to be constantly "fighting fires," senior management must ensure that marketing initiatives are adequately evaluated and that the foundation for evaluation is built into the project. This chapter highlights the importance of evaluating marketing activities and the critical role of the administrator in that process.

WHAT IS EVALUATION AND WHY IS IT IMPORTANT?

Evaluation involves the systematic assessment of the efficiency and effectiveness of a marketing initiative. The evaluation of a marketing campaign can be simple or complex, depending on the nature of the campaign. If the evaluation effort is well thought out, however, it should follow a straightforward, logical path.

Evaluation is an essential component of the marketing plan, and its functions include monitoring the progress, measuring the efficiency, and determining the effectiveness of the initiative. The evaluation process provides certain checks and balances to the process, helping to ensure that deadlines are met, budgets are adhered to, and the project otherwise stays on track.

Ultimately, the marketing effort will need justification, and this requires an adequate evaluation effort. The evaluation process allows for midcourse corrections and provides insights that should be useful in developing the next marketing initiative. The gist of each evaluation effort should be a set of lessons learned that can be applied to future projects.

Despite its importance, evaluation is anathema to many marketers. The artsy, creative work and the thrill of the marketing hunt are what excite marketers, not the evaluation "scut work" carried out after the fact. A marketer's conception of what is really important to the organization may differ from that of management, and the marketer's direct involvement in marketing activities may cause them to focus on the details while management is more interested in the big picture. For these reasons, senior management must take an active role in managing the evaluation effort. Marketing staff may be justifiably consumed with the promotional campaign du jour, but senior management must keep matters in the proper perspective. Evaluation can and should serve as a useful tool for management.

EVALUATION AS A MANAGEMENT TOOL

The feedback obtained through evaluation efforts can serve to inform management in a variety of ways. Information collected might include the following:

- the effectiveness of marketing in general;
- the effectiveness of the particular technique;

- the relative significance of marketing among other critical success factors;
- the quality of the marketing department or the outside agency;
- the perception of the public with regard to the organization;
- the reactions of competitors and collaborators; and
- program strengths, weaknesses, and areas in need of improvement.

WHO CARES ABOUT EVALUATION?

Senior management (including marketing management) should care more about the evaluation of marketing campaigns than anyone else. After all, they are the ones who will be judged (and presumably rewarded) based on the effectiveness of the marketing effort. This doesn't mean that marketing staff is not interested in feedback, but the perspective of management should be different.

Many other stakeholders may have an interest in successful promotional efforts. Staff members within the organization clearly have an interest in the impact of promotional activities. Feedback from the evaluation effort provides an appreciation of the type of response that may be anticipated from the public and the expectations customers will bring with them. Members of the organization's board of directors have a clear interest in the quality of the marketing effort, not just for its results but for what it says about the organization.

Funding agencies such as foundations (not for profit) or investors (for profit) have an interest in the effectiveness of marketing from their respective positions. Even government agencies funding a demonstration project or research effort may have a vested interest in how effectively the project was promoted.

Finally, colleagues in both healthcare and marketing are likely to have an interest in the effectiveness of various marketing techniques.

Other healthcare organizations may hope to benefit from your experience, and other marketers may consider applying a successful technique in another setting.

CHALLENGES TO EVALUATION IN HEALTHCARE

Intrinsic to healthcare are many unique challenges to the evaluation of marketing efforts. At the institutional level, the healthcare organization may have unclear, competing, and diffuse goals. A large hospital or a health system is likely to be pursuing a number of goals simultaneously, and whatever marketing resource the organization utilizes will likely be faced with promoting multiple goals, some of which may actually conflict with each other.

Healthcare organizations (especially not-for-profit entities) often have different criteria for success than organizations in other industries. The bottom line may not be the ultimate measure of success, managers may be more accountable to the trustees in terms of the quality of care provided. Indeed, healthcare organizations may knowingly operate programs at a loss on the assumption of indirect benefits above and beyond any profit generated directly from that program.

A number of intangibles may be involved in measuring success for a healthcare organization. True, patient volume, revenue, and profit margin should be considered, but less concrete benefits, such as visibility, market presence, patient satisfaction, or spin-off referral potential, may be equally important. The difficulty involved in placing a value on these intangibles only complicates the situation.

Efforts that contribute to enhancing the organization's status in the community or its relationship with other entities have a value attached to them, as do efforts that cast a negative light on the organization. The challenge, of course, is to place a dollar value on such activities.

These challenges do not mean that administrators should not try to evaluate their marketing efforts. But they do demand aggressive and creative approaches to evaluation that take these factors into consideration. These challenges can be converted into opportunities by documenting the benefits marketing brings to the organization above and beyond any contribution to the bottom line.

PLANNING FOR EVALUATION

Every marketing plan should include an evaluation plan that lays out the process for assessing the initiative. An accounting of effort should be made relative to success achieved. At the beginning of each marketing cycle, planning future efforts is essential. At the end of each cycle, the success of the combined effort must be evaluated. Regardless of the nature of our marketing efforts, we must have a way to keep score, otherwise we're back to "Ready, Fire, Aim" marketing. Without the aiming part of the equation we are really just taking expensive potshots at the marketplace.

The evaluation plan should follow the same steps outlined in Chapter 3 for marketing planning. Building evaluation into the marketing plan ensures that evaluation will start where it is supposed to—at the very beginning. The evaluation of a marketing initiative should be top of mind from the outset of the process and, in fact, should be built into the process itself. Goals and objectives should be specified on the front end, and this process should involve the marketing resource. The standard against which the effort will be measured should be known from the beginning of the project so that activity can be focused on specified results. Delaying the evaluation process to the end of the project limits the ability to compare intended results with actual results.

Some aspects of evaluation must be addressed before, during, and after implementing the campaign. Pretests may be performed at the outset and posttests at the end. The assumptions made about the project, the concepts formulated, and the objectives specified should be stated with eventual evaluation in mind. Indeed, the implementation component of the marketing plan can actually serve as the worksheet for evaluation activities.

The evaluation plan should

- lay out the process for evaluation;
- determine what is to be evaluated;
- identify the appropriate methods for evaluation;
- specify the types of data that will be required and how these will be obtained; and
- set the time lines for completing the various types of evaluation.

Outside consultants may need to be employed to develop and implement the evaluation plan. In fact, in some situations using an outside evaluator may be desirable or even essential. Like marketing itself, evaluation is something of an art, and training in-house staff to become professional evaluators may not be cost-effective. Fees paid for evaluation consultants are likely to be dollars well spent, and the arrangement will ensure that an objective evaluation of the initiative will be undertaken.

TYPES OF EVALUATION

Evaluation involves two major types of analysis: process analysis and outcome analysis. For our purposes, outcome analysis is separated into short-term outcomes and longer-term effects. In addition, cost analyses and ethical evaluation should be part of the process.

The best evaluation technique to implement depends on what is being evaluated, so effective evaluation must take into account the marketing approach. The challenge is to pick an evaluation technique that accurately assesses the specific type of marketing activity. An experienced evaluator can design measurement tools that will work with a particular media plan or segmentation strategy. For instance, if the campaign relies heavily on television and broadcast advertising, a broad community-based sample is required to measure the impact of the message. If the implementation has relied on direct mail, then the measurement approach must target those same consumer segments. A media plan driven by an ongoing PR activity calls for measurement that accounts for "column inches" placed in publications and "minutes of air time" accumulated through broadcast outlets.

Once an effective measurement tool is in place, stick with it. Since change in the relative positions of the organization compared to its competition is being measured, measuring the same things in the same way with similar questions is important. This way, changes identified reflect changes in attitudes or behavior and not changes in the methodology employed.

QUESTIONS TO ASK IN EVALUATING THE MARKETING CAMPAIGN

In assessing the success of a marketing campaign a number of questions should be raised. These include:

- How appropriate was the message for the target audience?
- How effective were the channels utilized?
- How well did the message reach the target audience?
- What changes resulted from the communication initiative?
- To what extent did the campaign achieve its goal(s)?
- Did the initiative engender any negative unintended consequences?
- Were the benefits derived from the exercise worth the cost of doing it?

Process Evaluation

Process evaluation assesses systems, procedures, communication processes, and other factors that contribute to the efficient operation of a marketing initiative. Process evaluation is used to document how well a program has been implemented and includes both concurrent monitoring and retrospective analyses. This type of evaluation is used to examine the operations of a program, including which activities are taking place, who is conducting the activities, and who is reached through the activities.

Process evaluation assesses whether resources have been allocated or mobilized and whether activities are being implemented as planned. It involves ongoing monitoring of the processes employed, including benchmarks and milestones to assess along the way. It examines both the mechanics of the process and the substantive content of the effort.

Process evaluation includes an assessment of whether messages are being delivered appropriately, effectively, and efficiently; whether materials are being distributed to the right people and in the right quantities; whether the intended program activities are occurring; and any other measures of how well the program is working.

Outcome Evaluation

Outcome evaluation is used to assess the effectiveness of a marketing campaign in meeting its stated objectives. While process evaluation considers how well the process is carried out, outcome evaluation considers the consequences (intended and unintended) of the campaign. The outcome evaluation plan is developed during the planning phase as a basis for identifying changes that did or did not occur as a result of the program. This type of evaluation assesses the results of the program and determines whether the program has achieved its outcome objectives.

The key measurement areas to track include awareness of the product, advertising awareness and recall, knowledge level, attitudes and perceptions, images of product and users, experience with the product, and behaviors (trial and repeat). Questions specific to the particular product or campaign should be asked of the target audience at this stage in addition to the earlier, general questions about attitudes and behaviors regarding the topic.

The following points should be kept in mind as the outcome evaluation is developed:

- The design should be appropriate for the particular marketing activity.
- Baseline measures should be established for tracking changes related to desired outcomes.
- The activity should be evaluated in accordance with specified outcomes and time frames.
- The degree of scientific rigor should be appropriate to the project.
- Change should be measured against marketing objectives and not against the program's goal.
- Progress toward outcomes should be measured even though objectives may not be completely met.

The timing of outcome evaluation is an important consideration, since the findings from the evaluation will differ depending on the point at which measurement occurs. For example, if several exposures to a message are required before those targeted take action, sufficient implementation time should be allowed to achieve the intended level of exposure. If immediate action is expected after exposure, then outcome measurement should take place soon after the promotional effort. If effects are not expected for at least a year, outcomes should not be measured until then.

Keep in mind that any marketing initiative is likely to generate unintended consequences. These consequences may be positive or negative but either way they may create a "monster" that is hard to control once released. On the positive side is the risk of generating more business than can be accommodated or creating the impression that the organization has more capabilities than it really has. On the negative side is the risk of attracting patients who are not really candidates for the service, alienating physician partners, or evoking an aggressive response on the part of a competitor. While anticipating each and every consequence of an activity is impossible, serious thought must be devoted to this topic during the planning phase. This process can be facilitated by examining each objective in turn for the potential consequences of achieving that objective.

Patient activity data, increased phone calls, increased donations, or increases in the volume of business in the areas being promoted can be critical indicators. The best way to capture these indicators is to look at both the internal (actual volume) data and external (consumer perception) data.

Impact Evaluation. Impact evaluation determines the extent to which the marketing campaign actually induced the desired change. While outcome evaluation is more focused on specific effects of the initiative, impact evaluation examines the broader effects and looks at changes that really make a difference.

To this end, impact evaluation is likely to consider the impact of the initiative on the target audience, on the organization, and on the community. The impact is quite different if members of the target audience become aware of a service as a result of promotional efforts or if they actually change their behavior as a result of the initiative. For the organization to receive increased inquiries concerning the service indicates a different result than if it experiences increases in volume. Exposing members of the community to HIV/AIDS education is quite different than seeing the incidence of new HIV cases decline.

Information generated through impact evaluation informs decisions on whether to expand, modify, or eliminate a particular policy or program, and can be used in prioritizing actions. In addition, impact evaluation assesses the effectiveness of programs and services by addressing the following questions:

- Did the initiative achieve the intended goal?
- Can the initiative explain the impact, or is the impact the result of some other factors?

- Does the impact of the program vary across different groups of intended audiences and geographic areas, and over time?
- Does the initiative have any unintended effects, either positive or negative?
- How effective is the program compared with alternative interventions?

Cost Analyses

Increasingly, health professionals are being asked to justify a marketing initiative in terms of its ROI. Some type of financial analysis should be conducted before the project begins and every effort made to track the benefits that accrue to the organization (in terms of visibility, perception, market share, volume, and revenue) as a result of the marketing activity. Not only does this task require a carefully constructed marketing plan, but it also demands detailed record keeping with regard to both the expenditures and revenues associated with a marketing initiative.

The costs associated with a program can be measured through either a cost-benefit analysis or a cost-effectiveness analysis. A cost-benefit analysis is a systematic cataloging of effects as benefits (pros) and costs (cons), valuing those effects in monetary units, and then determining the net benefits of the proposed project or activity relative to the status quo (net benefits equals benefits minus costs). Some cost analysis can take place concurrently with the campaign, but most of it will occur after the campaign has been completed and enough data have been collected to gauge the results of the campaign. (This is another area where it might be worthwhile to obtain outside expert input.)

A cost-effectiveness analysis may be used to assess the comparative effects of expenditures on different health interventions. Therefore, defining the core concepts of "effectiveness" is necessary. A very simple definition of effectiveness in health-related activities is that health services are considered effective to the extent that they achieve health improvements in real practice settings. A cost-effectiveness analysis requires a numerical estimate of the magnitude of the effects of an intervention on desired outcomes. This is usually expressed in a cost-effectiveness ratio, which is the difference in effectiveness between an intervention and the alternative.

Unlike most other industries, healthcare may embark on initiatives that are not profitable in the normal business sense. Evaluation techniques can still be used even when it is not possible to place a dollar value on everything. Thus, cost-effectiveness analysis can and should take into consideration the intangible aspects of the service-delivery process in its evaluation.

A number of things make ROI measurement a challenge in healthcare marketing. Among these are the time delay in the appearance of marketing results and the fact that the use of health services is not likely to be triggered by marketing but rather is situational. Further, many efforts toward marketing health services simply don't have a measurable return, even when accounting capabilities are present. Ultimately, a variety of factors are likely to influence the use of health services. As a result, other measurements (market share, brand position, preference, etc.) are likely to have more validity (and measurability) in the long run than does ROI.

The best measures of ROI in healthcare are softer measures like goodwill, awareness, and public relations coverage. If marketing efforts raise brand awareness (and, thus, brand equity) by a certain number of percentage points, this is a rough indicator of ROI. While healthcare organizations are beginning to look more closely at ROI measurement techniques, they still have a long way to go in adopting techniques from other industries.

Ethical Evaluation

Marketing initiatives should be subjected to an ethical evaluation—and this is particularly important in healthcare. A number of different concerns have been raised over the years related to claims made for health-related goods and services, the endorsement of various products, and the marketing activities of health professionals and organizations. As a result, various legal constraints have been put into place.

Ultimately, however, the ethical principles of the healthcare organization must maintain the integrity of the marketing campaign. As noted elsewhere, there is a bond of "trust" between healthcare providers and their customers, and the dependent relationship that patients have with clinicians makes them particularly vulnerable to misleading claims. All marketing should reflect professionalism and healthcare marketing should emphasize integrity and honesty in advertising. Certainly, any marketing should be appropriate for the organization and should be an accurate reflection of its mission.

The promotion of healthcare organizations must avoid misleading or exaggerated claims and not offer inappropriate incentives for the use of services. Celebrity endorsements should be factual and be able to support the claims that they make on behalf of the organization. The marketer may not have the same perspective as senior management when it comes to decisions on marketing ethics, and every effort should be made to keep everyone on the same page. This is another area in which involving the organization's administration is likely to be crucial.

HOW TO EVALUATE THE MARKETING DEPARTMENT

Often those in senior management are not experienced enough in marketing to assess the effectiveness of the marketing resource that is utilized. They may not be in a very good position to determine the quality of work the marketing resource is doing. Often, the marketing department itself participates in evaluating and reporting on the effectiveness of its own initiatives. While internal and external evaluation can examine the quality of the marketing campaign, assessing the quality of the marketing resource is up to senior management.

Whatever marketing resource is chosen should

- display an attitude of teamwork with senior management;
- prepare actively for interaction with the management team;
- adhere to the schedule and stay within budget;
- remain vigilant with regard to unintended consequences;
- keep the organization's mission in mind;
- operate in accordance with specified goals and objectives;
- display ethical and professional behavior;
- take the initiative in developing promotional efforts;
- effectively market itself to the organization and "teach" marketing to others; and
- emphasize results over appearances.

CRITICAL SUCCESS FACTORS

- Build evaluation into every marketing activity.
- Use evaluation of marketing activities as a marketing tool.
- Have a well-thought-out evaluation plan.
- Understand the different types of evaluation.
- Appreciate the nature of ROI in healthcare and be able to realistically measure it.
- Maintain ongoing management involvement in the marketing evaluation process.

CHAPTER 9

Healthcare Marketing: A Survival Strategy

Now that we have covered just about everything you need to know about healthcare marketing, we come to the most important question: How can the administrator use marketing to ensure the success of the organization? This chapter summarizes the role of the healthcare executive as it relates to the organization's marketing function and examines the implications of marketing for the ultimate success of the organization.

THE CHANGING STATUS OF MARKETING

Just as healthcare continues to change, so does the nature of healthcare marketing. The changes that have been taking place in the role of marketing are worth recounting, since the nature of marketing determines the relationship of management to the endeavor. These changes mean that the relationship between administrators and marketing today is considerably different than it was just a few years ago.

Looking back at the state of healthcare marketing, it was not long ago that healthcare administrators gave little thought to the marketing function. If marketing was implemented at all, it was a minor function that existed outside the framework of the organization.

With the exception of inherent marketing activities, such as networking and communication, marketing activities were typically outsourced, peripheral to the operation of the organization, and worthy of only limited resources. Marketing was a "passive" activity from the perspective of the organization.

Although formal marketing activities increasingly gained acceptance, marketing still remained in the "Oh, by the way…" category. Marketing remained primarily a minor outsourced task that had no direct relationship to the organization or its operation. Even if marketing activities were performed internally, they remained a "necessary evil" relegated to some out-of-way area of the hospital. *If money was budgeted for marketing, the amount was generally miniscule, and the marketing staff was certainly not allowed anywhere near the management team. Marketing services were essentially "ordered out," and nothing more was expected from the marketing resource than to see that ads ran in a timely fashion and within budget.

As healthcare organizations began to appreciate the value of marketing, a niche—albeit small—was carved out for the marketing staff. While still a "fringe" operation, the marketing function was at least moved under the umbrella of the organization to a greater extent. The uses to which marketing resources could be put expanded in the minds of administrators, although few within senior management interacted directly with the marketing resource. The resources made available to marketing staff were increased, and more contact was allowed with other departments. Even at this point, however, marketing activities typically remained reactive rather than proactive.

As these activities found greater acceptance, marketing came to be recognized as a legitimate function—and a worthwhile investment—for the healthcare organization. Marketing departments were established, senior marketing professionals were recruited, and someone from administration was given responsibility for overseeing this function. In many cases, progressive administrators actually became champions for marketing. Marketing came to be included as a line item in the organization's budget, along with funding for staff, promotional activities, and support services. Marketers gained increased autonomy and, while they may not have been contributing to the strategic direction of the organization, they continued to expand their role.

Over time, marketing came to be more of a "cabinet-level" department, with the marketing director accepted as part of the management team. Additional resources were allocated for marketing activities, and marketers became more proactive within the organization. Administrators began to seek the input of marketers on the front end, rather than simply assigning a task to them after the project was already under way.

In the final stage of this progression, the marketing director was brought to the table with the rest of senior management, perhaps even in the role of a vice president for marketing. At this point, the marketer was in a position to provide input into strategic planning, directly influencing the decision-making process, rather than waiting around for marching orders. Even more important, marketing was finally helping to drive the organization rather than vice versa. The strategic plan was being formulated based on input from marketing, making the organization increasingly consumer driven.

This progression followed by marketing has required the administrator to become increasingly involved with marketing activities. Marketing has been drawn from the outer reaches of the organization into the inner circle, making marketing as important as accounting, purchasing, human resources, or operations. Indeed, marketing has become *more* important since information generated through the marketing effort should guide the strategic direction of the organization. The administrator now seeks input from the marketing staff, and the marketer should be consulted for just about anything outside the walls of the organization (and many things inside).

As will be seen in this chapter, the changed status of marketing within the healthcare organization has introduced new responsibilities for management in relation to this function. Not only can the marketing function not be ignored, but virtually every decision must be made within the context of the marketing endeavor.

THE ROLE OF MARKETING IN THE ORGANIZATION

The ultimate purpose of marketing is not to sell things but to manage the reputation and grow the business of the organization. Growing the organization includes a wide range of activities but essentially represents expanding business opportunities and increasing the volume of business. Few services in healthcare sell themselves, and the marketer must take the lead in promotional activities. The enhanced role of marketing reflects its importance for the growth and success of the organization.

Some would argue that the primary function of marketing is to link the organization with its customers. Potential customers typically find out about the organization and its services through the marketing effort. The decision to use a service is likely to be influenced by the marketing effort. The creation of a loyal customer is likely to depend heavily on the effectiveness of internal marketing. Marketing should define and personify the organization and link it to critical audiences both inside and outside the organization.

To a great extent, the marketing department is the eyes and ears of administration. While most departments and managers are focused inward, the marketing department is primarily focused outward. The marketing staff is constantly interacting with customers and potential customers, obtaining feedback from the general public, and testing ideas in the marketplace. Marketing staff are in the best position to determine what promotion is likely to work best with a particular audience and to identify the issues that may be associated with a particular promotional effort. The marketing staff should be constantly on the lookout for a better way to promote the organization and should remain vigilant with regard to the business development opportunity that lurks around the corner.

The marketing department should also serve as the voice of senior management. It has the communication tools and expertise needed to support the corporate mission, strategy, and tactics, and it allows administration to eloquently present its case.

Perhaps above everything else, marketers should be seen as catalysts for change. No department in any enterprise is as dedicated to the analysis and pursuit of change as marketing. As such, marketers do more than just lubricate the machinery of the modern healthcare organization, they are vital to the generation of advances in medicine, new technology, new entrepreneurial entities, and new products and services that will make a difference in people's lives. The marketing effort should spark a response in potential customers and spur the organization on to even better customer service.

Marketing is also the organization's primary resource for meeting the competition. Effective marketing is essential for the organization to compete in today's marketplace. The marketing effort should have a direct impact on visibility, image, volume, market share, revenue, and any number of other measures of success. In a consumer-driven market, "packaging" is critical, and this is where the marketing resource can differentiate the organization from its competitors.

THE ROLE OF THE MARKETING DIRECTOR

If we are to concede that the primary functions of marketing are enhancing the organization's reputation and contributing to its growth, this implies a very different role for the marketing director than might be thought. From this perspective, the marketing director's responsibilities extend far beyond the everyday management of the marketing department, and it has implications for internal and external relationships. The role of the marketing director is broader and deeper given this scenario.

First and foremost, the marketing director should be the direct liaison with management. Senior management and the marketing director should operate in lockstep as they seek to advance the organization. The marketing director should be a constant source of new ideas and approaches and provide support for the organization's strategic plan.

The marketing team must also share responsibility for integrating marketing into the framework of the organization. Healthcare organizations are not comfortable including marketing within the "inner circle," and marketers are not used to being integrated into a complex healthcare organization. While much of the impetus for integration must come from senior management, the marketing director must play a key role in successfully integrating this function into a potentially hostile structure.

The marketing director should be prepared to contribute to the strategic direction of the organization. This means not only staying on top of the overall marketing plan and specific marketing initiatives, but also developing an understanding of the organization's strategic approach and the role that marketing plays in its implementation. Given that information generated through the marketing effort is critical to determining the future direction of the organization, the marketing director should anticipate challenges and opportunities and regularly present them to senior management.

Through all of this, the marketing director must actively support marketing team building and must constantly sell the marketing function to the organization's administration. The first rule of marketing is that the marketer should sell *himself.* The healthcare administrator will not automatically think of marketing when it is time to make a strategic decision. Thus, it behooves the marketing director to maintain a presence to ensure that marketing is allowed appropriate input.

Healthcare organizations are not known for their innovative approaches to marketing. They often look like a school of fish, all making similar adjustments at the same time as they react to trends and new buzzwords. The marketing director has chief responsibility for sorting through the promotional options available and ensuring that the organization is contemporary but unique in its marketing approach. The marketing director should keep up with marketing trends in other industries and be prepared to adapt them to healthcare.

Finally, the marketing director must be proactive in evaluating the effectiveness of any marketing initiatives. Most healthcare administrators do not have marketing backgrounds or know how to statistically evaluate marketing activities. As tedious as they may perceive the evaluation process to be, the marketing director should ensure that appropriate evaluation mechanisms are put into place to measure the effectiveness and efficiency of every marketing activity.

THE ROLE OF SENIOR MANAGEMENT

One of the points made throughout this book is that marketing is too important to be left to marketers. This doesn't just refer to the role of administration in directing the marketing effort but to the multifaceted interaction between administration and marketing—indeed, the incorporation of marketing into the framework of the organization.

Only senior management can orchestrate the inclusion of marketing into the "inner circle." It is not enough to ask for respect for the marketing department; the skids have to be greased in order to ensure full integration. This does not only refer to structural integration but also to philosophical integration. Effective managers find a way to get the concept of marketing embedded into the DNA of the organization.

With marketing, as with other aspects of the organization, senior management must provide the big picture. Most healthcare professionals—and this includes marketers—are so buried in the trenches that they have a hard time seeing the forest for the trees. The administrator must be able to not only maintain the larger perspective but also to convey it to the marketing staff.

At the same time, the marketing department is likely to be the most active interface with the outside world. Management must get used to the idea of consulting with the marketing team whenever a decision must be made. If the marketing director is doing her job, the director should be prepared to assess the situation in light of the marketplace and offer useful input with regard to strategic direction.

Senior management must ensure that marketing has appropriate input and makes its rightful contribution to strategic direction. Many within the organization will dismiss marketing as tangential to operations. After all, marketers are not clinicians. Senior management has the responsibility of ensuring that the marketing function is fully integrated into the organization, that marketing has access to all appropriate parties within the organization, that marketing is allowed to provide adequate input, and that the marketing function operates in sync with other functions within the organization.

Management must ensure that the infrastructure necessary to make the marketing effort successful is in place. This means more than a budget for staff and office space and includes support for data acquisition and analysis, primary research, and professional development. Further, it means that the marketing staff has access to all relevant departments and professionals and that all necessary information is freely available to them.

Finally, senior management is responsible for overseeing the marketing evaluation effort. Marketing staff are likely to have some capabilities with regard to evaluation, especially given their likely experience with marketing research. However, evaluation will not be top of mind for professionals who are trying to meet promotional deadlines. Additionally, marketers are not likely to appreciate the significance of evaluation to the organization's big picture, nor are they likely to have expertise in measuring ROI. Senior management must take an active role in evaluating the effectiveness and efficiency of the marketing effort. Senior management, not the marketing staff, will ultimately have to justify marketing expenditures and outcomes.

In the final analysis, the manager must *become* a marketer—not in the sense of developing marketing campaigns but in terms of thinking and acting like a marketing manager. As noted earlier, marketing must be embedded in the DNA of the organization, and this can only be accomplished by senior management. Every associate of the organization must become a marketing representative, and this is not something that the marketing department can bring about. Further, only senior management can ensure that the marketing resource has appropriate input into strategic decision making and that any marketing plan faithfully reflects the organization's image and strategic thrust.

QUESTIONS CEOS SHOULD ASK ABOUT THE IMPACT OF THEIR MARKETING EFFORTS

- Why are we doing marketing anyway?
- What is our marketing strategy? Do we have one?
- How is marketing contributing to the overall strategic direction of the organization?
- Are our marketing efforts turning every employee into a marketing representative?
- Are our marketing efforts contributing to a better understanding of the market and its needs?
- How are our marketing efforts contributing to brand enhancement?
- Are our marketing efforts capturing the relationship or just the sale?
- Can we determine the unintended consequences of our marketing efforts, especially the negative ones?
- Are our marketing efforts anticipating the changes taking place in healthcare—that is, are they positioning us for the healthcare environment of the future?

- Do our marketing efforts have a cumulative effect on our position within the market or do each stand alone?
- Am I taking an active role in marketing efforts or leaving critical decisions to marketers?

CONCLUSION

Throughout the book, we have repeatedly noted the importance of teamwork to the success of the marketing function—particularly the interface between senior management and the chosen marketing resource. A team effort is essential for the organization to be successful at marketing and to continue to grow. Both senior management and marketing have responsibilities in this regard, and undesirable results are likely unless both parties live up to their responsibilities. This relationship must involve mutual respect, mutual benefits, and symbiotic cooperation if the marketing endeavor is to be successful.

CRITICAL SUCCESS FACTORS

- Understand how developments in healthcare, technology, and the marketing craft influence the organization's approach to promotions.
- Appreciate the role of the marketing function within the organization.
- Understand the role of the marketing director.
- Understand the role of senior management in relation to marketing.
- Track the impact of the organization's marketing on an ongoing basis.

About the Authors

RICHARD K. THOMAS, PH.D., has been involved in market research and marketing in the healthcare field for more than 30 years. He is a principal in Health and Performance Resources and provides consultation to a wide range of healthcare organizations. He holds an associate professor appointment in the Department of Preventive Medicine at the University of Tennessee and has published extensively on healthcare topics. He was previously the editor of *Marketing Health Services*, a publication of the American Marketing Association.

MICHAEL CALHOUN has 30 years of experience in marketing, communications, and public relations. He began his career in financial services marketing and transitioned into healthcare marketing in the 1980s. He spent 12 years as the chief marketing officer for one of the nation's largest healthcare systems and has subsequently been involved in strategic marketing management and corporate communications in a variety of settings. He has applied healthcare marketing principles as a marketing director, public relations director, media relations trainer, corporate spokesperson, executive speechwriter, and communications consultant.